AF822540

Regenerative Medicine

By

Prof, Dr. Patrick Treacy

Copyright

Copyright © 2025 Patrick Treacy

Published by

BookFuel™

All rights reserved. No part of this book may be reproduced or transmitted in any form or by any means, electronic or mechanical, including photocopying, recording, or by any information storage and retrieval system, without written permission from the publisher and author.

Dedication

To the patients who placed their trust in me, to the colleagues and mentors who shared their wisdom, and to the future generations of doctors and scientists who will carry this work far beyond my reach. This book is also dedicated to the quiet resilience of those who heal — not only in body, but in spirit — and to the idea that within every cell lies the promise of renewal.

Acknowledgement

No book, like no scientific advance, is the work of one person alone. I owe an enduring debt of gratitude to the teachers who inspired curiosity in me, the colleagues and researchers around the world who have collaborated with generosity, and the countless patients who have, knowingly or not, taught me what healing truly means.

I would like to thank the many institutions and organisations that have supported my research and clinical work over the years, and the international congresses that have given me a platform to share ideas — from IMCAS in Paris to the World Regenerative Medicine Congress at King's College London. My sincere thanks also go to those who have recognised my efforts through awards and invitations to lecture; these honours belong as much to the teams and patients who made the work possible as they do to me.

To my family and friends, whose patience and encouragement sustained me through long hours and endless revisions, I offer heartfelt appreciation.

Finally, to the pioneers — past, present, and yet to come — who continue to push the boundaries of regenerative medicine, I acknowledge your courage and your imagination. We each play only a small part in a much larger story, one that will long outlive us, and I am grateful to have added even a few lines to its opening chapters.

Contents

Q1 – What is Bioregenerative Medicine?

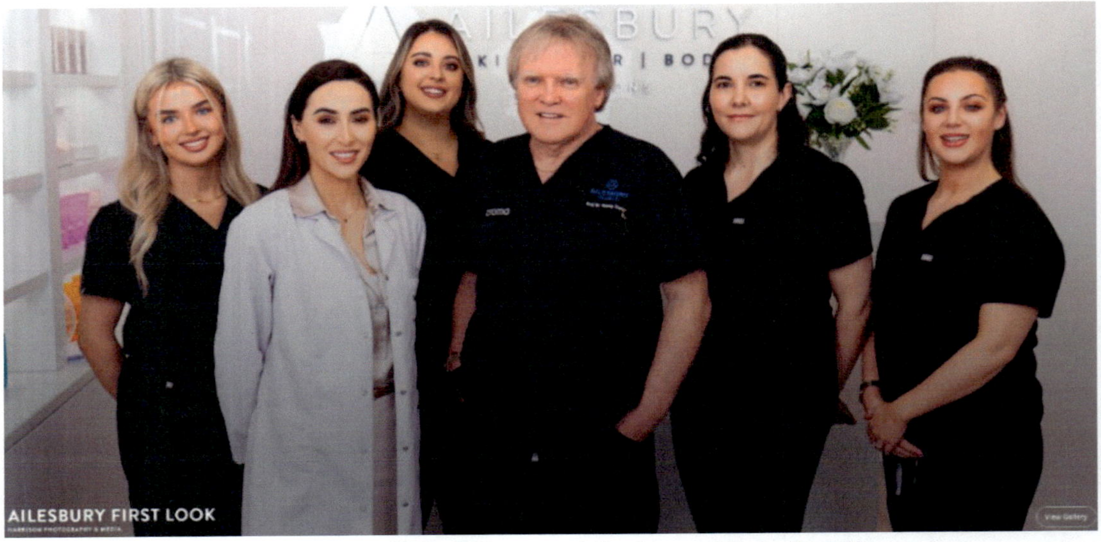

Bioregenerative Medicine Team – Ailesbury Clinic Dublin

Bioregenerative Medicine represents a transformative leap in biomedical science, harnessing the body's innate capacity to repair and regenerate damaged tissues and organs. This dynamic field integrates stem cell biology, tissue engineering, and advanced biomaterials to develop innovative therapies that address conditions ranging from chronic wounds to organ failure. By focusing on the body's own repair mechanisms, enhanced through scientific innovation, bioregenerative medicine offers hope for curative treatments that could reduce dependence on traditional surgeries and lifelong medications.

At its core, bioregenerative medicine employs cell-based therapies, utilizing stem cells—whether embryonic, adult, or induced pluripotent—to stimulate tissue repair or regenerate functional tissue. Induced pluripotent stem cells, in particular, have revolutionized the field by allowing adult cells to be reprogrammed into a pluripotent state, thereby sidestepping ethical concerns associated with embryonic stem cells and minimizing the risk of immunological rejection.

Complementing these cellular approaches, tissue engineering designs biocompatible and biodegradable scaffolds that provide a framework for cells to grow and mature into functional tissue. These scaffolds are often combined with growth factors such as VEGF or TGF-β, which guide and enhance the regenerative process, ensuring seamless integration with the patient's tissues.

The therapeutic potential of bioregenerative medicine spans multiple medical disciplines. In orthopaedics, for example, stem cell injections and biomaterial scaffolds are used to repair bone defects, cartilage lesions, and ligaments, offering less invasive solutions for injuries that once required surgery. In dermatology, cell-based dressings and engineered skin substitutes accelerate healing in chronic wounds and burns, significantly improving outcomes for patients with complex injuries. Cardiovascular applications focus on repairing heart tissue after myocardial infarction and enhancing vascularization in ischemic tissues, while neurological research explores stem cells and biomaterial implants to treat central nervous system injuries and neurodegenerative diseases.

Perhaps most ambitiously, bioregenerative medicine aims to reconstruct entire organs using lab-grown tissue grafts, which could alleviate the global shortage of donor organs available for transplantation.

Technological advancements underpin these therapeutic strides. The advent of 3D bioprinting enables the creation of patient-specific tissue structures, layer by layer, potentially revolutionizing organ repair and replacement. Exosomes and extracellular vesicles—tiny, cell-derived particles—are being investigated for their role in intercellular communication, promoting tissue repair and reducing inflammation. Meanwhile, gene-editing tools such as CRISPR/Cas9 allow precise correction of genetic abnormalities, enhancing the regenerative potential of cells prior to transplantation. These innovations, born from multidisciplinary collaboration across molecular biology, materials science, and bioengineering, are propelling bioregenerative medicine toward a future in which personalized, precision therapies become the standard of care.

Despite its promise, bioregenerative medicine faces significant challenges. Ensuring the safety and efficacy of these therapies requires rigorous preclinical and clinical evaluation to establish standardized protocols and minimize risks. Ethical and regulatory frameworks are evolving to balance innovation with patient safety, particularly concerning stem cell use and gene editing. The high cost of advanced regenerative therapies also presents a barrier, highlighting the need for scalable manufacturing processes and healthcare policies that improve accessibility.

Nevertheless, as clinical trials advance and produce positive outcomes, the field is poised to broaden its indications and gain wider global acceptance. Bioregenerative medicine aligns closely with the shift toward personalized medicine, tailoring treatments to each patient's unique genetic and physiological profile. Its potential to deliver definitive, curative interventions positions it as a cornerstone of future medical practice.

As research continues to mature, bioregenerative therapies could redefine how diseases are approached, offering solutions that not only heal but also restore the body's natural vitality. For patients and practitioners alike, this field heralds a new era of medicine—one in which regeneration is not just a possibility, but a transformative reality.

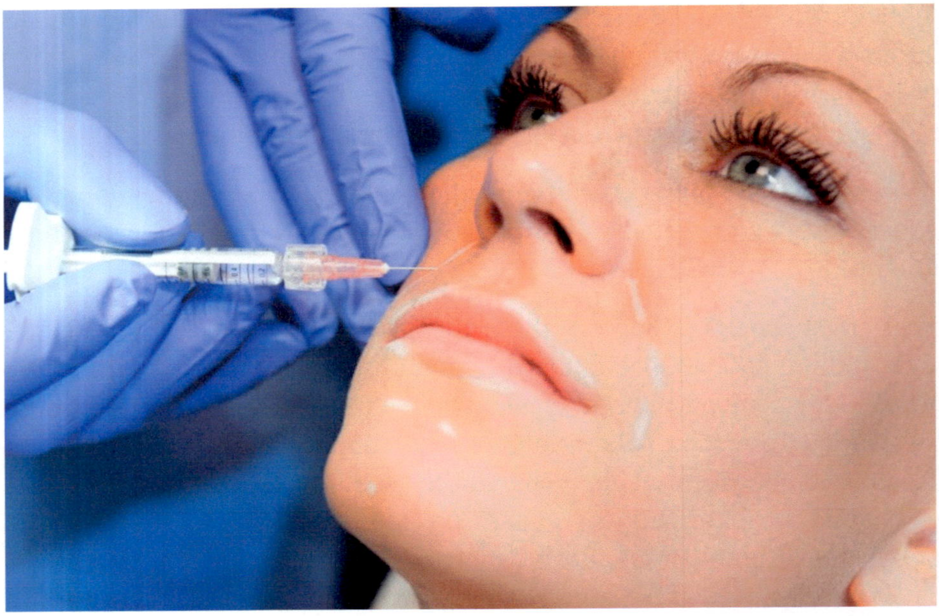

Q2 – What is a eukaryotic cell?

A eukaryotic cell is a type of cell that contains a true nucleus enclosed by a nuclear membrane and membrane-bound organelles such as mitochondria, the endoplasmic reticulum, Golgi apparatus, and, in plant cells, chloroplasts. This compartmentalization allows eukaryotic cells to carry out specialized functions within distinct organelles, enhancing efficiency and complexity compared to prokaryotic cells, which lack a nucleus and most membrane-bound organelles. Eukaryotic cells constitute all multicellular organisms—including animals, plants, and fungi—as well as certain single-celled organisms like protists.

At the core of bioregenerative and aesthetic medicine lies a deep understanding of cellular processes, particularly those involving eukaryotic cells and their intricate systems for communication and material transport. Eukaryotic cells, which form the foundation of multicellular life such as animals, plants, and fungi, as well as some single-celled protists, are distinguished by their complex internal architecture. Unlike prokaryotic cells, which lack a defined nucleus, eukaryotic cells possess a true nucleus enclosed by a nuclear membrane, along with specialized membrane-bound organelles including mitochondria, endoplasmic reticulum, Golgi apparatus, and chloroplasts in plant cells.

This compartmentalization enables eukaryotic cells to perform highly specialized functions with remarkable efficiency, making them essential to the advanced regenerative processes utilized in aesthetic medicine. Within these cells, a sophisticated network of endosomal compartments plays a pivotal role in sorting, trafficking, and processing materials, laying the groundwork for innovations such as exosome-based therapies.

Q3 – Tell me about Bioregeneration in Aesthetic Medicine?

Regenerative medicine holds significant potential across various facets of aesthetic medicine, particularly in areas such as hair restoration, skin rejuvenation, genital enhancement, and facial and body contouring. Below, I outline the key applications where regenerative techniques—including platelet-rich plasma (PRP), stem cell therapies, exosomes, and growth factors—are most effective. These treatments focus on promoting tissue repair and rejuvenation with minimal invasiveness. Here, I will examine the main areas of potential within aesthetic medicine.

1. Hair Restoration

Regenerative medicine is highly effective for treating hair loss conditions such as androgenetic alopecia by stimulating follicle regeneration. Platelet-rich plasma (PRP) injections deliver targeted growth factors to the scalp, enhancing hair thickness and density. Additionally, stem cell therapies—particularly those utilizing adipose-derived stem cells—improve follicle health and reduce inflammation. This approach is widely used to address pattern baldness in both men and women, providing a non-surgical treatment option with low risk and promising results in hair regrowth.

2. Skin Rejuvenation

This is a broad area where regenerative medicine excels in addressing aging, texture concerns, and skin damage. Treatments such as PRP facials, stem cell-infused creams, and exosome therapies stimulate collagen production, reduce wrinkles, fade scars—including acne scars—and improve skin elasticity and barrier function. These methods are particularly effective for anti-aging, hyperpigmentation, and accelerating wound healing. Often, they outperform traditional fillers or laser treatments by promoting long-term skin health. Additionally, topical regenerative products are becoming increasingly popular for daily skincare use.

3. Genital Rejuvenation

Regenerative techniques are increasingly used to enhance both function and appearance in intimate areas. For women, the O-Shot involves injecting platelet-rich plasma (PRP) into the clitoris and vaginal walls to improve lubrication, sensitivity, arousal, and orgasm intensity. It also addresses issues such as urinary incontinence and vaginal laxity caused by aging or childbirth. For men, the P-Shot consists of PRP injections into the penis to enhance erectile function, increase firmness and size perception, and improve sensitivity. This treatment is often used to help with erectile dysfunction and Peyronie's disease.

In addition, stem cell therapies can support tissue regeneration, improve skin smoothness, and reduce discomfort during intercourse. These procedures are minimally invasive and utilize the patient's own cells or blood, reducing the risk of adverse reactions.

4. Facial Rejuvenation

Beyond general skin care, regenerative medicine specifically targets facial aesthetics by using platelet-rich plasma (PRP) or stem cells to restore volume, smooth wrinkles, and minimize scars caused by acne or surgery. It is especially effective for treating under-eye hollows, nasolabial folds, and enhancing overall facial radiance. These treatments are often combined with microneedling to improve the absorption of growth factors, maximizing their rejuvenating effects.

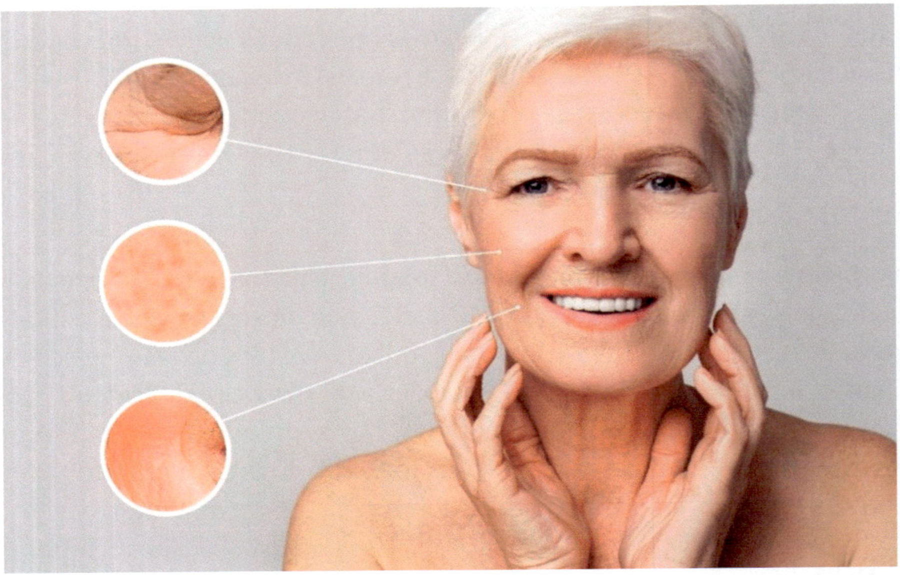

5. Body Contouring and Soft Tissue Enhancements

Regenerative techniques, such as adipose-derived stem cell-enriched fat grafting, are used for natural augmentation in areas like the breasts, buttocks, or hands. These methods help restore lost volume caused by aging or weight loss while simultaneously improving skin quality and graft survival. This approach offers a more natural alternative to synthetic fillers.

In summary, the strength of regenerative medicine in aesthetic applications lies in its ability to harness the body's own healing mechanisms to achieve natural, long-lasting results with fewer side effects. However, outcomes can vary depending on factors such as age and overall health. These treatments continue to evolve as ongoing research advances the field.

The fusion of Bioregenerative Medicine and Aesthetic Medicine

The fusion of bioregenerative medicine and aesthetic medicine is transforming the pursuit of beauty by harnessing the body's natural ability to heal and regenerate. This emerging synergy combines advanced cellular therapies, growth factors, and biomaterials to enhance and maintain a youthful appearance, offering patients minimally invasive, biologically driven solutions. By leveraging the body's intrinsic repair mechanisms, these treatments not only address aesthetic concerns but also promote sustainable, natural-looking results, marking a new era in cosmetic care.

At the core of this convergence are cell-based therapies, such as stem cells, platelet-rich plasma (PRP), and exosomes, which stimulate tissue repair and regeneration. In aesthetic applications, these therapies promote collagen synthesis, improve skin elasticity, and encourage hair growth, delivering subtle yet transformative outcomes. Growth factors—including TGF-β, PDGF, VEGF, and FGF—play a pivotal role by driving cell proliferation, tissue repair, and angiogenesis. These molecules can be harnessed to accelerate healing and remodel tissues in targeted areas such as the face or scalp.

Complementing these approaches, advanced biomaterials like collagen or hyaluronic acid scaffolds provide structural support for new tissue formation, prolong the effects of regenerative therapies, and enable precise delivery of healing factors to treatment sites.

In clinical practice, bioregenerative techniques are revolutionizing aesthetic medicine across multiple domains. For skin rejuvenation, PRP—derived from the patient's own blood—is applied through microneedling or injections to stimulate collagen and elastin production. This reduces fine lines, wrinkles, and acne scars while improving overall skin texture. Exosome therapy, utilizing cell-derived vesicles rich in proteins and RNA, enhances tissue repair, hydration, and skin tone, offering a cutting-edge approach to rejuvenation.

In hair restoration, stem cell-derived products or PRP, often combined with scalp microneedling, activate hair follicles to promote thicker, fuller hair. For soft tissue volume restoration, fat grafting enriched with stem cells provides longer-lasting results compared to traditional methods, while biostimulatory injectables such as calcium hydroxyapatite or poly-L-lactic acid gradually improve skin quality by stimulating collagen production.

Scar reduction and wound healing also benefit from bioregenerative approaches. Growth-factor-rich topicals and regenerative dressings accelerate recovery and minimize scarring. Additionally, combining PRP with ablative or non-ablative laser treatments further enhances healing and collagen remodeling, optimizing aesthetic outcomes.

The advantages of bioregenerative therapies are significant, particularly due to their natural and autologous nature. Treatments such as platelet-rich plasma (PRP), derived from the patient's own blood or tissue, minimize the risk of allergic reactions and work in harmony with the body's intrinsic repair processes, producing gradual yet sustainable results.

However, challenges remain. Safety and efficacy rely heavily on standardized protocols, as variations in cell isolation methods, exosome purification, or growth factor concentrations can significantly impact outcomes. Thorough patient assessment is essential to manage expectations and identify any contraindications. The regulatory landscape varies globally; some cell-based therapies require extensive clinical data for approval, which can slow their adoption. Additionally, the high cost of novel regenerative treatments may limit accessibility, though advancements in technique and scalability have the potential to reduce costs over time.

Looking ahead, the integration of bioregenerative and aesthetic medicine holds immense promise. Advances in genomics and proteomics will enable personalized treatments tailored to an individual's genetic profile, optimizing regenerative outcomes. Combining regenerative products such as stem cells or exosomes with energy-based devices—like lasers or radiofrequency—may enhance results while minimizing downtime.

Ongoing research continues to refine the sourcing, concentration, and delivery of regenerative components, promising greater efficacy and consistency. Beyond current applications in skin rejuvenation and hair restoration, bioregenerative methods may soon address broader aesthetic concerns, including stretch marks, cellulite, and even functional aspects of aging tissues, thereby expanding the scope of aesthetic medicine.

The convergence of bioregenerative and aesthetic medicine is redefining how clinicians approach beauty, shifting the focus from superficial corrections toward biologically driven renewal. From PRP to exosomes and beyond, these therapies offer innovative, minimally invasive pathways to achieving aesthetic goals.

As research progresses and techniques evolve, practitioners and patients can anticipate increasingly refined, effective, and personalized approaches that not only enhance appearance but also harness the body's remarkable capacity for regeneration.

Q4 – Tell me about Exosomes and Aesthetic Medicine?

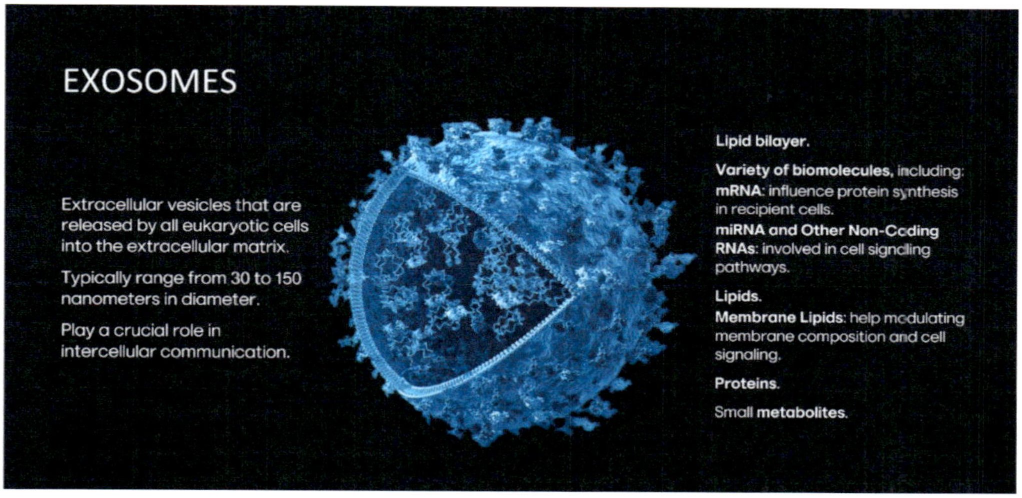

Exosomes, tiny extracellular vesicles secreted by virtually all cell types, are emerging as a groundbreaking tool in aesthetic medicine, offering a cell-free approach to skin rejuvenation, hair restoration, and tissue repair. Measuring just 30–150 nanometres in diameter, these vesicles originate within endosomal compartments called multivesicular bodies before being released into the extracellular environment through fusion with the cell membrane. Encased in a protective lipid bilayer, exosomes carry a rich cargo of proteins, lipids, and nucleic acids—including mRNA and microRNA—that enable critical cell-to-cell communication. By delivering molecular signals that influence recipient cell behavior, exosomes hold immense potential to enhance aesthetic outcomes through biologically driven regeneration.

In aesthetic medicine, exosomes exert their effects through multiple mechanisms that align seamlessly with the goals of rejuvenation and repair. They modulate cellular behavior by stimulating collagen production, promoting angiogenesis, and accelerating cell turnover—processes essential for revitalizing skin and supporting wound healing. Certain exosomes also exhibit anti-inflammatory and antioxidant properties, which can reduce post-procedure inflammation and oxidative stress, thereby enhancing recovery after treatments such as microneedling or laser therapy. In hair restoration, exosomes deliver growth-promoting signals to hair bulb cells, potentially reactivating dormant follicles and extending the anagen (growth) phase, leading to improved hair density and vitality. These multifaceted capabilities make exosomes a versatile tool for addressing a wide range of aesthetic concerns.

Clinically, exosome-based therapies are being integrated into aesthetic practice with promising results. For skin rejuvenation, exosomes can be applied topically or injected following procedures like microneedling or fractional laser treatments, allowing deeper penetration to improve skin texture, tone, and elasticity while accelerating recovery. In hair restoration, scalp injections of exosomes target thinning areas to support follicle health and promote thicker hair over time. Exosomes also excel in combination therapies, where they are paired with energy-based devices like radiofrequency or lasers, or with platelet-rich plasma (PRP), to amplify healing and regenerative effects. This synergistic approach enhances outcomes, making exosome therapy a valuable addition to the aesthetic clinician's toolkit.

The advantages of exosomes are significant, particularly their non-cellular nature, which simplifies their use compared to live cell therapies such as stem cell injections and reduces immunogenic risks. By modulating multiple signaling pathways, exosomes offer a comprehensive approach to tissue repair and regeneration. However, challenges remain in ensuring consistent quality and efficacy. The source of exosomes—whether derived from mesenchymal stem cells or other cell lines—along with their purity and concentration, varies widely among commercial products. Improper processing methods, including lyophilization or suboptimal storage, can damage the exosomal lipid bilayer, diminishing their bioactivity. Additionally, while early clinical results are promising, exosome-based treatments remain in the early stages of research and require more peer-reviewed studies and standardized protocols to confirm their safety and efficacy. Regulatory landscapes also vary globally, with some exosome products classified as experimental or subject to stringent guidelines for cell-derived therapies, necessitating careful navigation by practitioners.

The future of exosomes in aesthetic medicine is promising, with ongoing advancements poised to enhance their effectiveness and utility. Innovations in isolation techniques—such as tangential flow filtration and size-exclusion chromatography—aim to produce higher-purity exosomes with consistent dosing, thereby improving reliability in clinical applications. Researchers are also exploring ways to engineer exosomes with specific surface markers or customized cargo to more precisely target aesthetic concerns like deep wrinkles or resistant hair loss.

Hybrid therapies that combine exosomes with growth factors, peptides, or scaffold materials hold great potential to sustain and amplify their regenerative effects, opening new possibilities for achieving long-lasting results. As these developments progress, exosomes are set to play an increasingly prominent role in aesthetic practice.

Exosomes represent a transformative frontier in aesthetic medicine, offering a sophisticated, cell-free strategy to harness the body's regenerative potential. From rejuvenating skin and restoring hair to enhancing post-procedure recovery, these tiny vesicles are redefining the future of aesthetic care.

Plant-derived exosomes are immunologically well-tolerated and non-toxic, as noted in product presentations, supporting safe intravenous administration. Preclinical studies in cancers such as breast cancer have shown improved tolerance and efficacy using nano-encapsulated CBD delivered via exosomes.

Exosomes are nanosized (30–150 nm) lipid vesicles secreted by cells, carrying specific cargos like microRNAs (miRNAs) and proteins that enable targeted intercellular signaling. In contrast, secretomes encompass the full range of secreted molecules—including exosomes, microvesicles, and soluble factors such as cytokines—offering broader but less specific paracrine effects.

For example, exosomes derived from Centella Asiatica in products like "exo ox. intim" are isolated through complex methods such as ultracentrifugation to achieve purity and specificity, particularly for applications like CBD encapsulation. Meanwhile, secretomes are more easily collected as cell culture supernatants but are less pure and precise.

Overall, advancements in exosome technology and understanding continue to expand their therapeutic potential, positioning them as a key component in the evolving landscape of aesthetic and regenerative medicine.

Q5 – Tell me is there any difference in human, mammalian and plant derived exosomes?

Yes, there are notable differences between human-, mammalian-, and plant-derived exosomes, even though they share core characteristics as extracellular vesicles (EVs) involved in intercellular communication. These distinctions stem from their biological origins, molecular composition, modes of production, and therapeutic applications.

Similarities Across Exosome Types:

All exosomes are lipid bilayer–bound vesicles, typically ranging from 30 to 150 nm in diameter. They carry diverse bioactive cargos—including proteins, lipids, RNA, and DNA—that facilitate cell-to-cell signaling. Exosomes enable targeted delivery, protect their molecular contents from degradation, and participate in various physiological and pathological processes such as tissue regeneration, inflammation, and cancer progression. Let us now examine their origin and source.

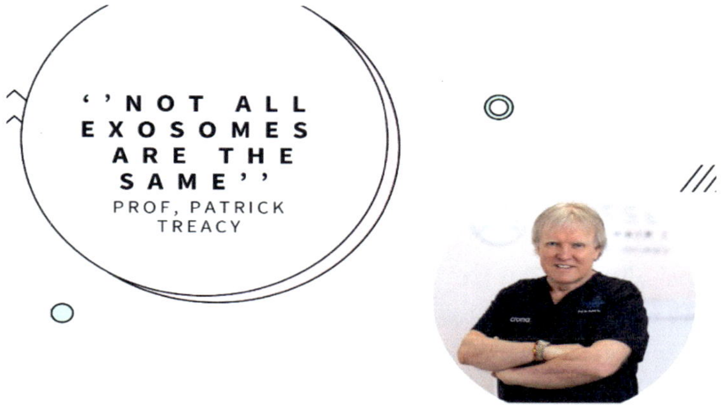

- ## Human-Derived Exosomes:
  - **Source**: Derived from human cells such as mesenchymal stem cells (MSCs), dendritic cells, and fibroblasts, obtained either from body fluids (e.g., blood, urine) or through cell culture systems.
  - **Example**: MSC-derived exosomes are widely studied for applications in regenerative medicine and cancer therapy.
  - **Relevance**: These exosomes are highly specific to human physiology, making them ideal for personalized medicine; however, their use is limited by donor variability, scalability issues, and ethical considerations.
- ## Mammalian-Derived Exosomes:
  - **Source**: Derived from non-human mammalian cells (e.g., bovine, murine, or porcine) or biological fluids such as bovine milk.

- **Example**: Bovine milk–derived exosomes have been investigated as nanocarriers for drug delivery, including cannabidiol (CBD) in neuropathy models.
- **Relevance**: These exosomes share structural and functional similarities with human-derived counterparts but are easier to obtain due to scalable sources like milk. They are widely utilized in preclinical research, although potential cross-species compatibility and immunogenicity issues remain challenges for clinical translation.

- **Plant-Derived Exosomes:**
  - **Source**: Isolated from plant tissues, juices, or cell culture systems (e.g., Centella asiatica in "Exo Ox. Intim," citrus, ginger, and cannabis).
  - **Example:** Centella asiatica–derived exosomes (7.5×10^{10} particles/mL) are utilized in regenerative gynaecology products.
  - **Relevance:** Sustainable, scalable, and cost-effective; plant-derived exosomes are increasingly used in cosmetic formulations (e.g., for skin rejuvenation) and in emerging therapeutic applications.

In terms of composition and cargo, human-derived exosomes contain human-specific proteins—such as tetraspanins (CD9, CD63, CD81)—along with microRNAs (miRNAs) and signaling molecules aligned with human physiological pathways, including growth factors like VEGF. The cargo profile reflects the donor cell's physiological or pathological state; for example, cancer-derived exosomes may carry oncogenic miRNAs, while mesenchymal stem cell (MSC)–derived exosomes are enriched with anti-inflammatory cytokines such as IL-10, promoting tissue repair and regeneration.

As noted in previous references to CBD and hyaluronic acid (HA), exosomes can encapsulate lipophilic compounds like cannabidiol (CBD) or be combined with HA for targeted delivery—an approach demonstrated in glioma models.

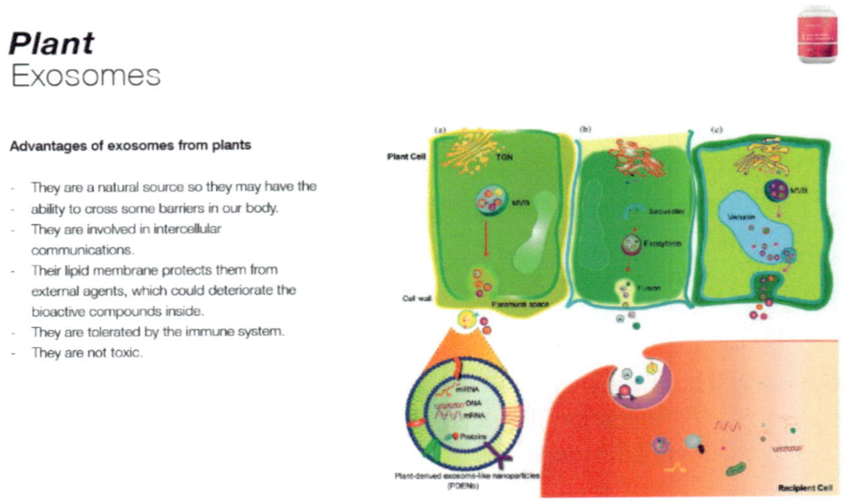

Mammalian-derived exosomes share many structural and functional similarities with human exosomes but exhibit species-specific surface markers (e.g., bovine CD63 homologs). They contain conserved cargos such as microRNAs (miRNAs) and proteins but often differ in their lipid composition. For instance, bovine milk–derived exosomes are rich in lactoferrin, making them suitable carriers for the oral delivery of compounds such as cannabidiol (CBD).

Plant-derived exosomes, on the other hand, contain plant-specific lipids, secondary metabolites (e.g., polyphenols), miRNAs, and proteins. For example, *Centella asiatica*–derived exosomes carry bioactive peptides and growth factors. Unlike mammalian or human exosomes, plant-derived exosomes lack animal-specific surface markers such as CD9.

In terms of **immunogenicity and safety**, human-derived exosomes demonstrate low immunogenicity when used autologously (derived from the same patient). However, allogeneic exosomes can elicit immune responses due to factors such as major histocompatibility complex (MHC) mismatches, and there is a potential risk of transferring pathogenic cargos (e.g., from cancer cells).

Mammalian-derived exosomes exhibit moderate immunogenicity because of cross-species molecular differences. Bovine milk exosomes, for example, are generally well tolerated but may cause mild immune reactions in sensitive individuals. Notably, milk-derived exosomes are classified as **Generally Recognized as Safe (GRAS)** by the U.S. Food and Drug Administration (FDA) for oral administration.

Plant-derived exosomes show the lowest immunogenicity among these types, as they lack animal-specific antigens. Exosomes derived from sources such as ginger or *Centella asiatica* have demonstrated no significant immune activation in *in vivo* studies.

Q6 – What are Autologous Exosomes?

Autologous exosomes are extracellular vesicles (EVs) derived from a patient's own cells—typically mesenchymal stem cells (MSCs), fibroblasts, or other somatic cell types—used for therapeutic purposes due to their roles in intercellular communication and tissue regeneration. These vesicles carry diverse bioactive cargos, including proteins, microRNAs (miRNAs), messenger RNAs (mRNAs), lipids, and metabolites, which facilitate cell-to-cell signaling and modulate physiological processes.

Among the various sources, MSC-derived exosomes are the most extensively studied because of their potent regenerative and immunomodulatory properties. Since autologous exosomes originate from the patient's own cells, they express self-antigens, thereby minimizing the risk of immune rejection or inflammatory reactions. This contrasts with allogeneic exosomes, which may provoke major histocompatibility complex (MHC)–mediated immune responses.

The molecular cargos of autologous exosomes reflect the physiological state of the donor cells, enabling them to promote natural repair and homeostatic mechanisms. For example, MSC-derived exosomes have been shown to attenuate inflammation and fibrosis in preclinical models of cardiac injury, osteoarthritis, and cutaneous wound healing.

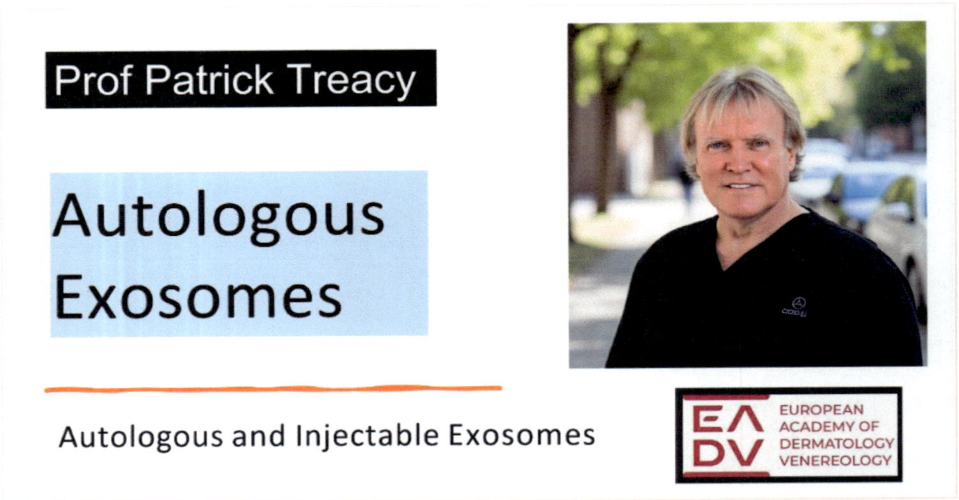

Author's cautionary note

Autologous mesenchymal stem cell (MSC) exosomes are considered safe for regenerative therapy due Due to their low immunogenicity and inherent compatibility with the patient's own biological system, autologous exosomes are considered highly biocompatible therapeutic candidates. However, their production remains both costly and technically complex. Autologous MSC-derived exosomes are obtained from a patient's own mesenchymal stem cells (MSCs), typically isolated from bone marrow, adipose tissue, or umbilical cord tissue collected during procedures such as biopsies.

Because they originate from the same individual, these exosomes express self-antigens—such as major histocompatibility complex (MHC) class I molecules—that minimize the risk of immune rejection or inflammatory responses. This contrasts with allogeneic (donor-derived) exosomes, which may provoke immune activation due to MHC incompatibility.

MSC-derived exosomes encapsulate a range of bioactive cargos, including microRNAs (miRNAs), growth factors (e.g., vascular endothelial growth factor [VEGF]), and anti-inflammatory cytokines (e.g., interleukin-10 [IL-10]), reflecting the regenerative and immunomodulatory properties of their parent cells. These vesicles promote tissue repair, angiogenesis, and immune regulation without eliciting adverse immune reactions.

Preclinical studies have demonstrated that MSC-derived exosomes can attenuate inflammation and fibrosis in models of cardiac injury, wound healing, and osteoarthritis.

Q7 – Can exosomes be mixed with other chemicals like CBD (cannabidiol) or HA (hyaluronic acid)?

Yes, exosomes can be combined with other bioactive compounds such as cannabidiol (CBD) or hyaluronic acid (HA), as supported by emerging scientific literature. Their lipid bilayer structure enables the encapsulation or surface association of both lipophilic molecules (e.g., CBD) and hydrophilic substances (e.g., HA), thereby enhancing stability, bioavailability, and targeted delivery. The following analysis summarizes key points from the provided product documentation and relevant studies, addressing the feasibility, mechanisms, and considerations of mixing exosomes with such compounds.

- **EXO POWDER:** Formulated with *Centella asiatica*–derived plant exosomes combined with 1% CBD. These exosomes (7.5×10^{10} particles/mL; 134.9–162.8 nm in size) are known to encapsulate and protect bioactive molecules such as growth factors and peptides—a capability that likely extends to CBD, given its lipophilic nature.
- **HA SOLUTION:** Comprises non-crosslinked hyaluronic acid enriched with amino acids including glycine, proline, lysine, and leucine. The application protocol involves mixing one vial of EXO POWDER with one vial of HA SOLUTION for topical or localized use in regenerative gynecology (e.g., vaginal revitalization).
- **Role of HA:** Enhances tissue hydration, elasticity, and collagen synthesis, thereby synergizing with the regenerative and reparative properties of exosomes.

Protocol

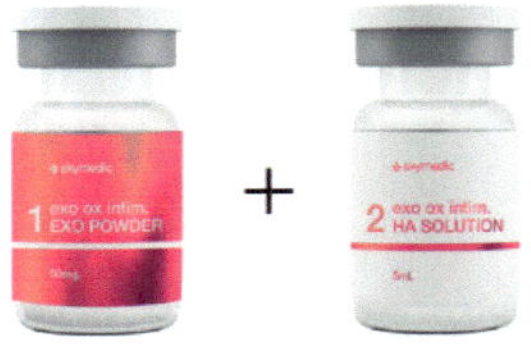

Use
Mix 1 vial of HA SOLUTION with 1 vial of EXO POWDER

Sessions
3 to 5 (may vary depending on individual patient differences)

Frequency
Every 3-4 weeks

Mixing with HA

Mechanism:

Hyaluronic acid (HA), a hydrophilic polysaccharide, is unlikely to be encapsulated within the lipid bilayer core of exosomes. However, it can be incorporated in formulations through solution mixing, surface association via electrostatic interactions, or chemical functionalization. HA is widely utilized in exosome-based products for skin and tissue regeneration. For instance, HA-functionalized exosomes have been shown to accelerate wound healing by enhancing tissue hydration and collagen synthesis. In dermatological applications, HA and exosomes are combined in formulations such as ExoCoBio's ASCE+ SRLV to improve skin hydration, elasticity, and repair—paralleling the Skymed "Exo Ox" product's intended role in vaginal rejuvenation. Additionally, studies demonstrate that exosomes suspended in HA-based hydrogels enable sustained release and improved therapeutic efficacy in tissue engineering and regenerative medicine contexts.

Benefits:

- **Complementary Effects:** HA's water-retention capacity and collagen-stimulating properties synergize with the regenerative and signaling functions of exosomes, aligning with the product's focus on restoring elasticity and hydration.
- **Stability of the Mixture:** Owing to its high biocompatibility, HA supports stable co-administration with exosomes, as reflected in the described formulation protocol. HA may serve as a carrier matrix, facilitating exosome retention and uniform distribution within target tissues.
- **Delivery Considerations:** While HA is typically co-delivered rather than encapsulated, its physicochemical characteristics—particularly molecular weight—can influence biodistribution and systemic delivery efficiency, necessitating formulation optimization for specific clinical applications.

Mixing with CBD

Cannabidiol (CBD), a hydrophobic compound, can be encapsulated within the lipid bilayer or internal lumen of exosomes, where it is protected from oxidative and enzymatic degradation and exhibits enhanced cellular uptake through endocytosis. Plant-derived exosomes, such as those from *Centella Asiatica*, are particularly well-suited for this purpose due to their natural capacity to encapsulate lipophilic bioactive molecules. CBD possesses anti-inflammatory, analgesic, soothing, and regenerative properties that complement the intercellular signaling and tissue-repair functions of exosomes.

Experimental studies have demonstrated that CBD-loaded exosomes—whether derived from plant or mammalian sources (e.g., cannabis or milk)—improve the bioavailability and therapeutic efficacy of CBD in models of cancer, neuropathy, and inflammation. For instance, camel milk–derived exosomes have been shown to protect CBD during oral administration, increasing its stability and absorption. Similarly, extracellular vesicles isolated from cannabis plants naturally contain CBD and can deliver it to target cells, promoting anticancer signaling pathways. Exosomes thus act as protective carriers, shielding CBD from premature degradation, as reflected in the product claim that their lipid membranes safeguard encapsulated compounds.

Mixing with Other Chemicals

Exosomes can also be combined with a range of bioactive compounds beyond CBD and hyaluronic acid (HA), depending on the intended application. Polyphenolic compounds such as curcumin, resveratrol, and quercetin, as well as peptides, miRNAs, and small-molecule drugs (e.g., metformin), can be encapsulated within exosomes or conjugated to their surface to enhance targeted delivery, stability, and therapeutic activity.

In regenerative and aesthetic medicine, exosomes are frequently integrated into polymeric matrices or nanomaterial systems—such as hydrogels or poly (lactic-co-glycolic acid) (PLGA) nanoparticles—to enable controlled or sustained release. These hybrid formulations improve local retention, promote gradual diffusion, and amplify regenerative outcomes in applications ranging from wound healing to skin rejuvenation.

Exosomes represent a promising, cell-free platform in aesthetic and regenerative therapies, with the potential to improve skin texture, support hair growth, and accelerate wound repair. However, their widespread adoption will depend on ongoing research, manufacturing standardization, and the establishment of regulatory frameworks to ensure product safety, consistency, and clinical efficacy.

Author's Cautionary Note

These formulations are intended for **topical or local administration**, not intravenous (IV) use. Systemic delivery—such as potential applications in glioblastoma (GBM)—requires rigorous evaluation of immune responses, biodistribution, and toxicity, as emphasized by medical experts concerned about mitochondrial effects. CBD's known potential to induce mitochondrial depolarization (via mPTP formation and increased reactive oxygen species) warrants caution. While exosomes may theoretically mitigate off-target effects through targeted delivery, there is currently no published data confirming this mechanism for the "Exo Ox" formulation.

Any combination of exosomes with pharmacologically active agents for systemic use should undergo comprehensive testing for purity, loading efficiency, release kinetics, and biosafety. At present, no exosome–drug formulations are clinically approved for systemic administration.

Evidence supports the feasibility of combining exosomes with **CBD (via encapsulation)** and **HA (via co-delivery)** to enhance stability, bioavailability, hydration, and regenerative outcomes in topical or gynecological applications. However, for systemic applications such as IV therapy in oncology, safety uncertainties—particularly regarding mitochondrial stability and immune tolerance—underscore the need for further preclinical validation. This aligns with the prudent skepticism expressed by Dr. Treacy. Detailed clarification of intended use (e.g., topical vs. systemic) and any additional chemical components would enable more targeted formulation recommendations.

Questions from the World Regenerative Medicine Congress 2025

(Kings College Cambridge University) to the author Prof Patrick Treacy by the audience of medical doctors and experts in their field

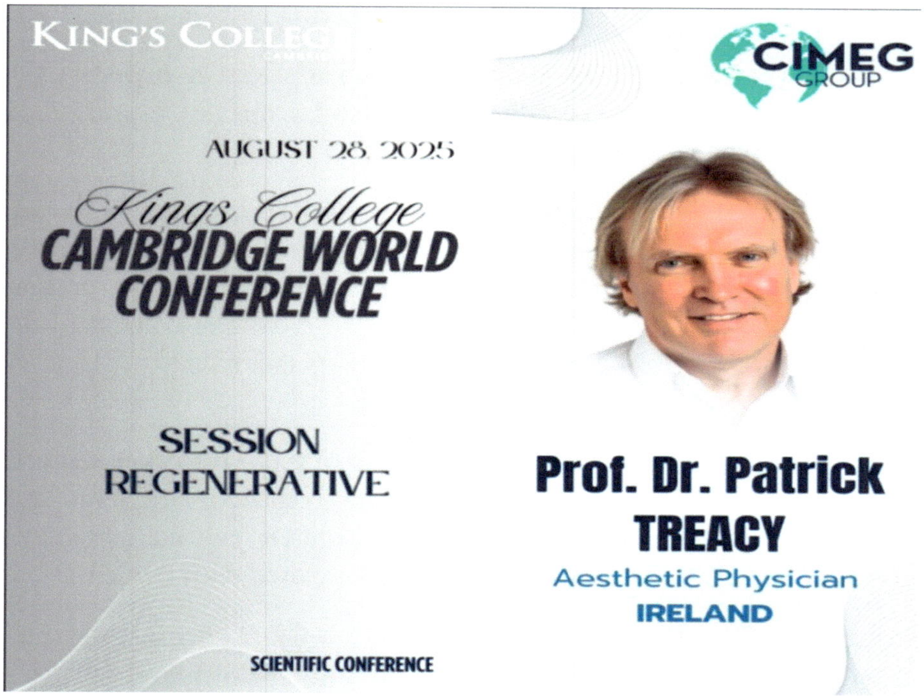

Audience Question: Do the exosomes and CBD operate independently, with their combined effects resulting from additive or parallel biological pathways without direct molecular interaction?

Authors answer: While independent activity is possible—such as exosomes promoting tissue regeneration through signaling molecules like growth factors, and CBD exerting anti-inflammatory and analgesic effects via the endocannabinoid system—current literature indicates that **synergistic interactions often surpass simple additive effects**. For example, CBD has been shown to modulate exosome biogenesis and release from cells, selectively inhibiting exosome secretion in cancer models to suppress tumor progression, while **exogenously applied exosomes enhance CBD's delivery efficiency and therapeutic impact**.

In the Skymed "Exo Ox Intim" formulation, CBD is described as complementing *Centella asiatica*–derived exosomes in tissue regeneration and repair. This suggests **parallel yet complementary mechanisms**, such as CBD's soothing effects on mucosal tissues operating alongside the exosomal stimulation of collagen synthesis and cellular renewal. However, the available documentation provides no direct evidence of molecular interaction between CBD and the exosomes within the formulation.

Experimental studies on CBD-loaded extracellular vesicles (EVs), including exosomes, demonstrate **enhanced anticancer efficacy** compared with either component alone—for instance, by sensitizing breast cancer cells to chemotherapy. Consequently, while independent action may occur in certain regenerative contexts, **functional synergy through interconnected biological pathways** is more frequently observed in therapeutic and experimental applications.

King's College Audience Question: Do the exosomes encapsulate or incorporate CBD within their vesicular structure, facilitating targeted delivery, cellular uptake, or modulated release via exosomal membrane fusion or endocytosis?

Authors answer: This represents a **primary mechanism underlying the observed synergy**. Exosomes are inherently suited to encapsulate lipophilic compounds such as CBD due to their lipid bilayer structure, which allows incorporation into either the vesicular lumen or the membrane itself. The *Centella asiatica*–derived exosomes featured in the product are noted for their ability to encapsulate and protect bioactive molecules—such as growth factors and proteins—a property that likely extends to CBD given its nonpolar characteristics.

Preclinical studies have demonstrated the **successful loading of CBD into exosomes**, resulting in improved delivery efficiency and pharmacological performance. Exosome-encapsulated cannabinoids exhibit **enhanced cellular uptake and targeted release** in cancer models, supporting their potential to amplify therapeutic outcomes compared with free CBD.

King's College Audience Question: Could this exosome-CBD combination be feasibly administered intravenously for the treatment of glioblastoma multiforme, considering factors such as blood-brain barrier penetration, tumour-specific targeting, immunological responses, and preclinical/clinical evidence supporting efficacy and safety?

Authors answer: Yes, this combination demonstrates **promising feasibility for intravenous (IV) application in glioblastoma (GBM)**, although current evidence remains primarily preclinical and not specific to *Centella asiatica*–derived exosomes. Exosomes possess an inherent ability to **cross the blood–brain barrier (BBB)** via receptor-mediated transcytosis, making them highly suitable for brain-targeted drug delivery—an advantage over free CBD, which exhibits limited BBB permeability.

Preclinical studies utilizing exosomes derived from brain endothelial or glioma cells have shown **efficient drug delivery to GBM sites**, validating their potential as nanocarriers for central nervous system therapies. CBD itself demonstrates **anti-glioma activity**, including inhibition of cellular energy metabolism, induction of apoptosis, and suppression of tumor growth. When combined with agents such as THC or standard chemotherapeutics, CBD exhibits **synergistic effects** in GBM models.

Encapsulation of CBD within exosomes further enhances these outcomes: recent formulations have achieved **greater cellular uptake and cytotoxicity in glioma cells**, outperforming free CBD. Moreover, CBD has been reported to modulate tumor-derived exosome release, thereby **reducing metastasis-associated signaling and improving overall therapeutic efficacy**.

However, significant challenges remain, including the **optimization of CBD loading efficiency**, **ensuring tumor-specific targeting** (e.g., through surface ligand modification), and the **need for GBM-specific in vivo and clinical studies** to confirm safety, biodistribution, and efficacy.

King's College Audience Question: What future research do you envisage for exosome-encapsulated CBD for gliomas?

Future research on **exosome-encapsulated CBD for glioma therapy** is strongly warranted. Although the *Exo Ox Intim* formulation is designed for localized application, its constituent components could conceptually inform the development of intravenous (IV) adaptations. However, such applications would necessitate rigorous **regulatory evaluation and clinical validation** prior to translation into systemic use.

In summary, the observed synergy most likely arises from **encapsulation (mechanism 3)** and **protection (mechanism 2)** mechanisms rather than from purely independent action (**mechanism 1**), indicating significant potential for future IV applications in GBM therapy. If additional information from the product manufacturer (e.g., Vytrus Biotech) or specific **exosome-loading protocols** becomes available, these hypotheses could be refined and experimentally validated.

Further discussion or experimental design development is encouraged. For instance, **CBD-loaded extracellular vesicles (EVs)** from diverse biological sources have been shown to facilitate **endocytosis-mediated cellular uptake**, thereby enhancing anti-tumor efficacy. Plant-derived exosomes, including those from *Centella asiatica*, demonstrate comparable capabilities, with reported high concentrations (e.g., 7.5×10^{10} particles/mL, as noted in the product presentation) that support efficient **cargo encapsulation and delivery**. This vesicular incorporation not only regulates **controlled release** but also markedly improves **bioavailability**, paralleling the performance of other nanoencapsulated CBD formulations.

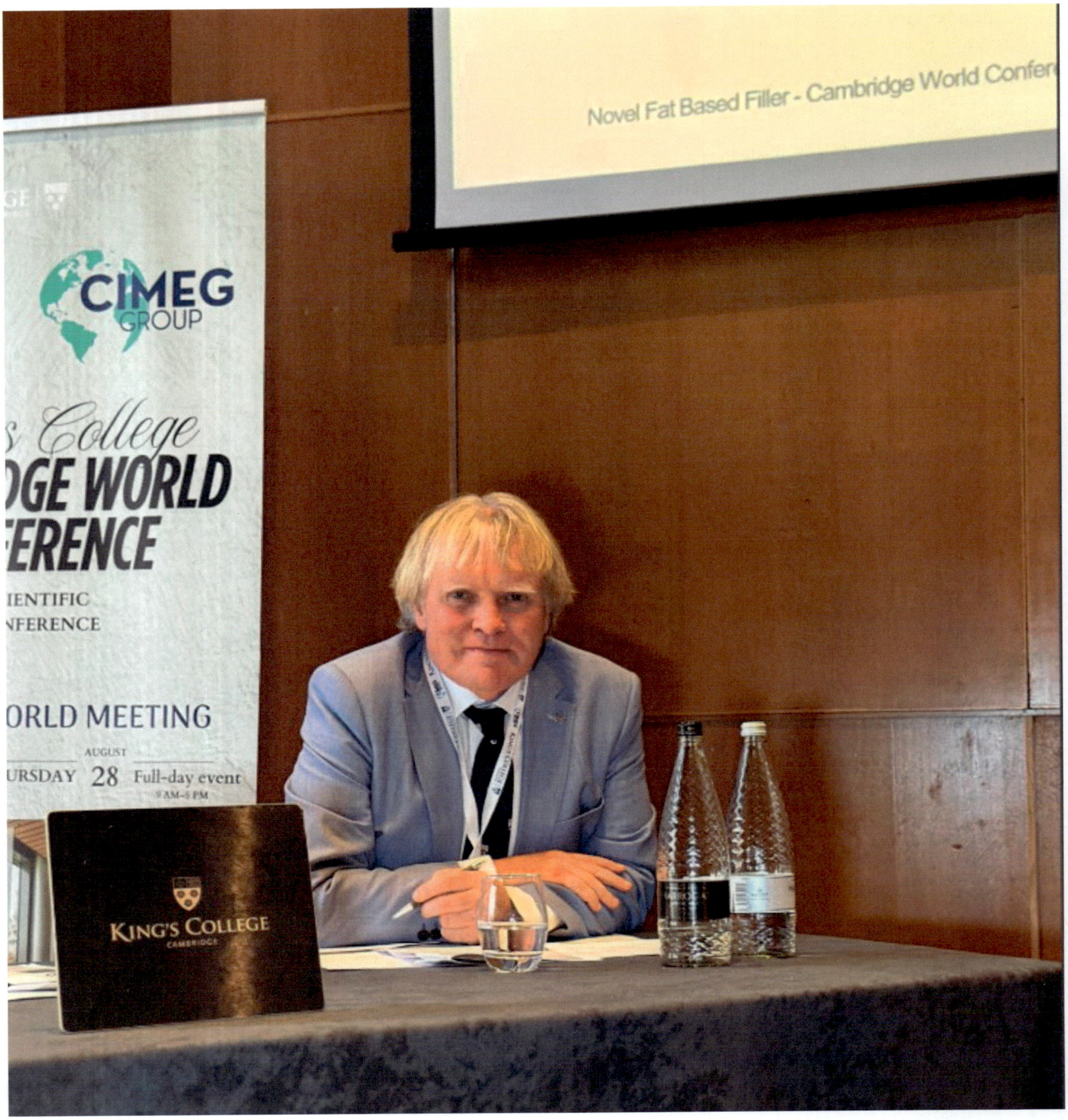

The author at the World Regenerative Medicine Congress Cambridge University

Q8 – What is an endosomal compartment of the cell?

An **endosomal compartment** refers to a network of membrane-bound organelles within eukaryotic cells that function in the **sorting, trafficking, and processing** of materials internalized through endocytosis or transported from intracellular sources such as the Golgi apparatus. Following endocytosis, external molecules or particles are enclosed within vesicles that fuse with **early endosomes**, which serve as the primary sorting hubs.

From there, cargo is directed along distinct pathways through intermediate compartments, including **recycling endosomes**, **late endosomes**, and in some cases, **multivesicular bodies (MVBs)**. This trafficking sequence determines whether internalized material is **recycled back to the plasma membrane** or **targeted to lysosomes for degradation**.

Collectively, endosomal compartments are critical for **maintaining cellular homeostasis**, **regulating receptor recycling**, and **controlling the processing and degradation** of proteins, lipids, and other macromolecules within the cell.

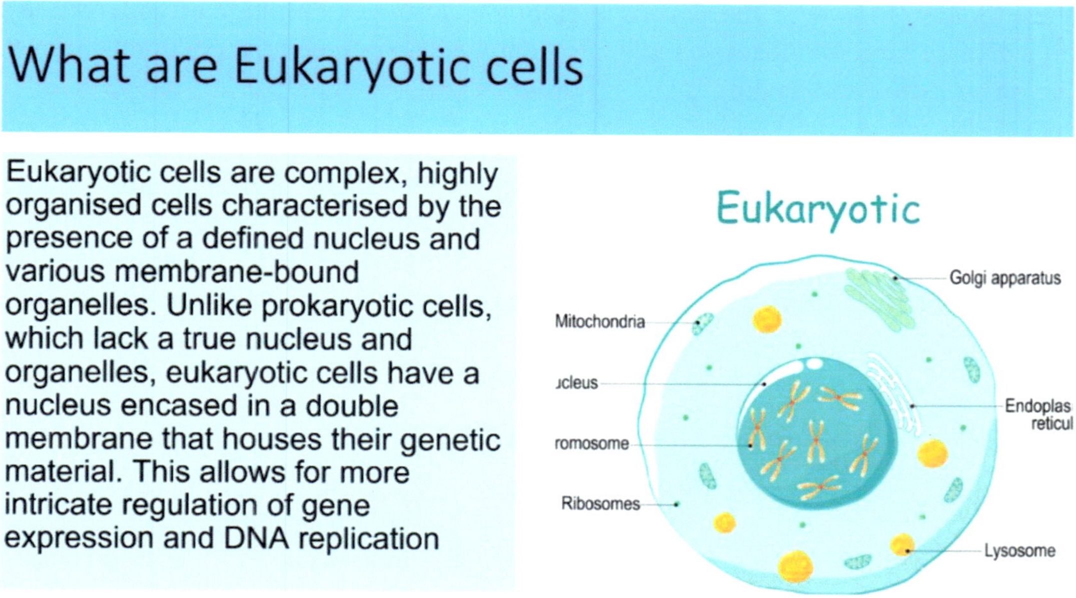

Q9 – What is Exosome cargo?

Endosomal compartments are a series of membrane-bound organelles within eukaryotic cells that regulate the **intake, sorting, and ultimate fate** of molecules internalized through endocytosis or transported from intracellular structures such as the Golgi apparatus. When external molecules or particles are engulfed at the cell surface, they are enclosed within vesicles that fuse with **early endosomes**, which function as the cell's primary sorting hubs. From there, the cargo may pass through **recycling endosomes**, **late endosomes**, or **multivesicular bodies (MVBs)**, each directing materials toward one of two principal fates: **recycling to the plasma membrane for reuse** or **delivery to lysosomes for degradation**.

This dynamic trafficking system is fundamental to **cellular homeostasis**, **receptor regulation**, and the **processing and degradation of proteins and other macromolecules**. In the context of **aesthetic and regenerative medicine**, endosomal compartments are of particular interest because they give rise to **exosomes**—nanoscale vesicles that are transforming approaches to tissue repair and rejuvenation.

Exosomes, typically measuring **30–150 nanometers** in diameter, are formed within **multivesicular bodies** of the endosomal pathway and released into the extracellular environment when these bodies fuse with the plasma membrane. Acting as **biological couriers**, exosomes transport a diverse cargo of bioactive molecules that mediate intercellular communication essential for tissue regeneration and healing.

Encased within a **lipid bilayer** enriched in **cholesterol and sphingomyelin**, exosomes safeguard a complex payload of **proteins, nucleic acids, lipids, and other signaling molecules**. Among their protein constituents are **growth factors** such as **VEGF, TGF-β, and FGF**, which promote cell proliferation, angiogenesis, and tissue repair, as well as **cytokines** like **IL-6** and **TNF-α**, which modulate immune responses and orchestrate tissue remodeling. Additionally, **enzymes and regulatory proteins** within exosomes influence **metabolic and signaling pathways**, further enhancing their regenerative and therapeutic potential.

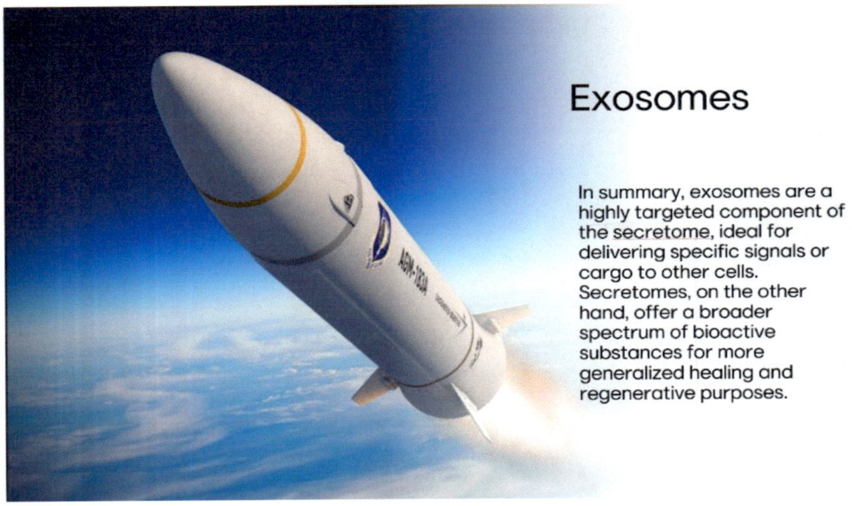

The **nucleic acid component** of exosomal cargo is equally pivotal, particularly in the realm of **aesthetic and regenerative medicine**. **Messenger RNA (mRNA)** molecules delivered by exosomes can be translated into functional proteins within recipient cells, thereby modulating cellular behavior to stimulate key regenerative processes such as **collagen synthesis**, **elastin production**, or **hair follicle activation**. Meanwhile, **microRNAs (miRNAs)**—small, non-coding RNAs that regulate gene expression at the post-transcriptional level—play crucial roles in governing **cell differentiation**, **proliferation**, and **apoptosis**, processes fundamental to tissue renewal and repair.

Depending on the **cellular origin** and **physiological context**, exosomes may also contain other RNA species, including **long non-coding RNAs (lncRNAs)** and **circular RNAs (circRNAs)**, which further refine gene expression networks in recipient cells. In some instances, exosomes encapsulate **DNA fragments**, **metabolites**, or **cell-adhesion molecules** on their surface, enabling **specific recognition and binding** to target cells. This molecular precision enhances their capacity for **targeted delivery** and **localized therapeutic action**, underscoring the expanding potential of exosomes as vehicles for **next-generation regenerative treatments**.

Q10 – What are the Functional implications of Exosome Cargo?

The **functional implications of exosomal cargo** are far-reaching, particularly in **aesthetic and regenerative medicine**, where these nanoscale vesicles drive **skin rejuvenation**, **hair restoration**, and **wound healing**. Through the transfer of their molecular payload, exosomes stimulate **collagen synthesis**, promote **angiogenesis**, and accelerate **cellular turnover**, resulting in improved **skin texture, tone, and elasticity**. Their intrinsic **anti-inflammatory** and **antioxidant** properties further support **post-procedural recovery**, helping minimize erythema, swelling, and downtime following interventions such as **microneedling**, **laser resurfacing**, or **chemical peels**.

In the context of **hair restoration**, exosomal cargo delivers **growth-stimulating biomolecules** that can reactivate **dormant follicles** and prolong the **anagen (growth) phase**, offering a promising, biologically based solution for patients with **thinning or weakened hair**. Beyond aesthetic applications, exosomes play pivotal roles in maintaining **tissue homeostasis**, **cellular communication**, and **immune modulation**. However, they also possess a **dual nature**—in pathological contexts, exosomes can propagate **disease-related signals**, contributing to processes such as **tumor growth**, **angiogenesis**, and **metastatic spread**.

The **integration of exosome-based therapies** into aesthetic practice depends on a deep understanding of **cellular biology**, particularly the dynamics of **endosomal compartments** where these vesicles originate. Despite growing enthusiasm, several **challenges** persist: establishing **standardized production and purification protocols**, ensuring **batch-to-batch consistency**, and navigating **complex regulatory frameworks** that govern clinical use. Ongoing advances in **exosome isolation**, **characterization**, and **bioengineering** are expected to enhance their **specificity**, **stability**, and **therapeutic potency**, paving the way for **personalized regenerative treatments**.

For aesthetic practitioners, exosomes represent a **next-generation therapeutic platform**—a means of **harnessing the body's intrinsic repair mechanisms** to achieve **natural, biologically driven rejuvenation**. Their emergence marks a paradigm shift in the concept of beauty, redefining it through the lens of **cellular regeneration and biological harmony**.

Q11 – What Are The implications of modifying the Exosome cargo?

Modifying the cargo of exosomes—the nanoscale vesicles secreted by cells that carry proteins, lipids, nucleic acids (such as miRNA and siRNA), and other bioactive molecules—has profound implications in **biomedicine**, particularly in **aesthetic and regenerative medicine**. By tailoring their molecular contents, exosomes can be engineered to amplify or redirect their natural roles in **cell-to-cell communication**, enabling advances in **drug delivery**, **disease modulation**, and **tissue regeneration**.

Enhanced Therapeutic Delivery and Efficacy:

Modifying exosomal cargo transforms these vesicles into **highly efficient, targeted delivery systems** for therapeutic agents. By incorporating specific **drugs, nucleic acids, or proteins**, engineered exosomes can protect sensitive molecules from enzymatic degradation in the bloodstream, **extend their circulation time**, and **enhance site-specific delivery** to target tissues. For instance, engineering exosomes with specialized **membrane proteins** can increase their cargo-loading capacity and improve intracellular delivery, facilitating **gene activation** or **protein expression** in recipient cells.

In aesthetic medicine, such modifications can enable exosomes to deliver **growth factors**, **miRNAs**, or **cytokines** that promote **skin rejuvenation**, **hair follicle activation**, or **tissue repair** in sensitive regions such as the **vaginal mucosa**. In regenerative contexts, cargo-engineered exosomes can enhance outcomes in **anti-ageing therapies**, **scar reduction**, and **cartilage repair** by delivering molecules that stimulate **cell proliferation**, **angiogenesis**, or **extracellular matrix remodeling**. Functionally, these interventions modify how exosomes interact with recipient cells, influencing key biological processes including **immune regulation**, **wound healing**, and even **oncogenic suppression**.

Innovative techniques—such as establishing **pH gradients** or using **electroporation**—have improved nucleic acid loading efficiency, allowing exosomes to transfer genetic material more effectively and modulate cellular behavior. These strategies can stimulate **collagen synthesis** for improved **skin elasticity**, enhance **vascularization**, and support **sexual wellness** by promoting **tissue regeneration** in genital applications.

Impact on Exosome Formation, Release, and Cellular Communication:

Altering exosomal cargo also influences their **biogenesis**, **secretion**, and **communication dynamics**. During formation within **endosomal compartments**, molecular sorting mechanisms determine which proteins, lipids, and RNAs are incorporated. Manipulating these pathways allows for **controlled secretion rates** and **customized cargo profiles**. For example, inhibiting certain enzymes can suppress exosome release, reducing the spread of pathological cargo in diseases such as cancer. Conversely, upregulating exosome secretion can be harnessed to enhance **regenerative signaling** in aesthetic applications.

In cosmetic and therapeutic contexts, fine-tuning exosomal cargo could optimize **delivery of regenerative factors** to specific targets—such as **hair follicles**, **fibroblasts**, or **neuronal cells**—to stimulate growth and repair. Additionally, **post-translational modifications** like glycosylation of RNAs or lipidation of proteins can refine how exosomes are packaged and transferred between cells, improving **target recognition** and **functional efficacy**. These engineered vesicles can transiently reprogram recipient cells by **boosting immune resilience**, **enhancing nerve regeneration**, or **modulating metabolic pathways**, outcomes that are particularly valuable in **facial rejuvenation** and **intimate health restoration**.

Applications in Aesthetic Medicine

In aesthetic medicine, **modified exosomes** represent a cutting-edge approach to regenerative treatment, offering targeted, biologically driven enhancement across multiple indications. Their ability to deliver customized molecular cargo—such as growth factors, cytokines, or nucleic acids—positions them as versatile tools for natural tissue restoration and rejuvenation.

- **Hair Restoration:** Engineered exosomes can deliver growth factors and signaling molecules that **reactivate dormant hair follicles**, stimulate dermal papilla cells, and enhance vascularization of the scalp. This leads to improved **hair density, thickness, and overall scalp health**, offering a promising solution for **androgenetic alopecia** and other forms of hair loss.
- **Skin Rejuvenation:** Cargo-loaded exosomes can promote **collagen and elastin synthesis**, accelerating skin renewal while reducing **wrinkles, scars, and hyperpigmentation**. Their anti-inflammatory and antioxidant properties further support post-procedure healing and enhance **skin radiance, firmness, and elasticity**, making them ideal adjuncts to treatments such as **microneedling, lasers, and chemical peels**.
- **Genital Rejuvenation:** Modified exosomes can improve **tissue hydration, sensitivity, and structural integrity** in intimate areas. By delivering regenerative molecules that stimulate **angiogenesis, collagen deposition, and nerve repair**, they can help address concerns such as **vaginal laxity, dryness, or erectile dysfunction**, contributing to enhanced **sexual wellness and comfort**.
- **Facial and Body Regeneration:** Exosomes can be tailored to support **volume restoration** and **tissue remodeling** in areas such as the **face, neck, or hands**. Unlike synthetic fillers, which merely add volume, exosome-based treatments promote **endogenous regeneration**, resulting in **natural, gradual, and long-lasting improvements** in contour and texture.

Challenges and Considerations

While the therapeutic potential of exosome modification is considerable, several challenges must be addressed before widespread clinical adoption. The **complexity of exosome biogenesis** makes **precise and reproducible cargo loading** difficult, and **off-target or unintended effects** may occur if natural exosomal signaling is disrupted. Ensuring **standardized isolation, purification, and characterization protocols** is critical to maintain consistency and safety.

From a **regulatory standpoint**, engineered exosomes occupy a gray area between biologics and nanomedicines, necessitating clear **guidelines for quality control, sterility, and ethical use**.

Clinically, treatment outcomes may vary depending on **patient-specific factors** such as age, hormonal status, metabolic health, and the integrity of local tissue environments. Furthermore, **long-term safety and efficacy data** remain limited, underscoring the need for **controlled trials and mechanistic studies** to validate their regenerative promise in aesthetic applications.

Q12 – Tell me about Growth factors?

Growth factors—naturally occurring proteins and peptides—act as the body's molecular architects, orchestrating essential cellular processes such as growth, proliferation, differentiation, and survival. Functioning as signaling molecules, they bind to specific receptors on target cells, initiating intricate cascades of intracellular events that shape cellular behavior. Their remarkable receptor specificity allows them to exert powerful biological effects even at low concentrations, amplifying signals through complex pathways that regulate functions ranging from embryonic development to tissue repair, immune modulation, and wound healing.

In aesthetic medicine, these biochemical messengers are redefining the boundaries of regenerative therapy. By leveraging the body's innate healing mechanisms, growth factors enable natural, biologically driven rejuvenation—supporting applications in **skin repair, hair restoration, and tissue regeneration**.

The diversity of growth factors reflects the complexity of their biological roles:

- **Epidermal Growth Factor (EGF):** Stimulates cellular proliferation and differentiation, particularly in epithelial tissues, making it a key driver of **skin repair and wound healing**.
- **Fibroblast Growth Factors (FGFs):** Support **angiogenesis, tissue regeneration, and embryonic development**, essential for maintaining dermal integrity and elasticity.
- **Platelet-Derived Growth Factor (PDGF):** Released during the clotting process, PDGF promotes **fibroblast and smooth muscle proliferation**, facilitating tissue reconstruction and scar remodeling.
- **Transforming Growth Factor Beta (TGF-β):** Regulates **cell proliferation, differentiation, and apoptosis**, playing a crucial role in **immune modulation** and **extracellular matrix synthesis**, which underpins collagen formation.
- **Vascular Endothelial Growth Factor (VEGF):** Drives **angiogenesis**, enabling the formation of new blood vessels that ensure adequate oxygenation and nutrient delivery during healing.
- **Insulin-Like Growth Factors (IGFs):** Promote **cell survival, growth, and metabolic balance** across various tissues, reinforcing regenerative capacity and homeostasis.

Each growth factor exhibits distinct yet complementary functions, underscoring their value in **targeted therapeutic applications**.

In aesthetic medicine, growth factors are integrated into advanced modalities such as **platelet-rich plasma (PRP)**, **topical formulations**, and **exosome-based therapies**, where they stimulate **collagen synthesis, enhance skin elasticity, and improve hair density**—yielding natural, long-lasting results. In wound-healing contexts, growth factors accelerate tissue repair by **recruiting fibroblasts, endothelial cells, and keratinocytes**, which contribute to **neovascularization, collagen deposition, and extracellular matrix remodeling**.

These regenerative properties make growth factors indispensable in both **corrective and preventive aesthetic treatments**, supporting faster recovery, improved skin texture, and enhanced overall tissue vitality following procedures such as microneedling, laser resurfacing, or surgical interventions.

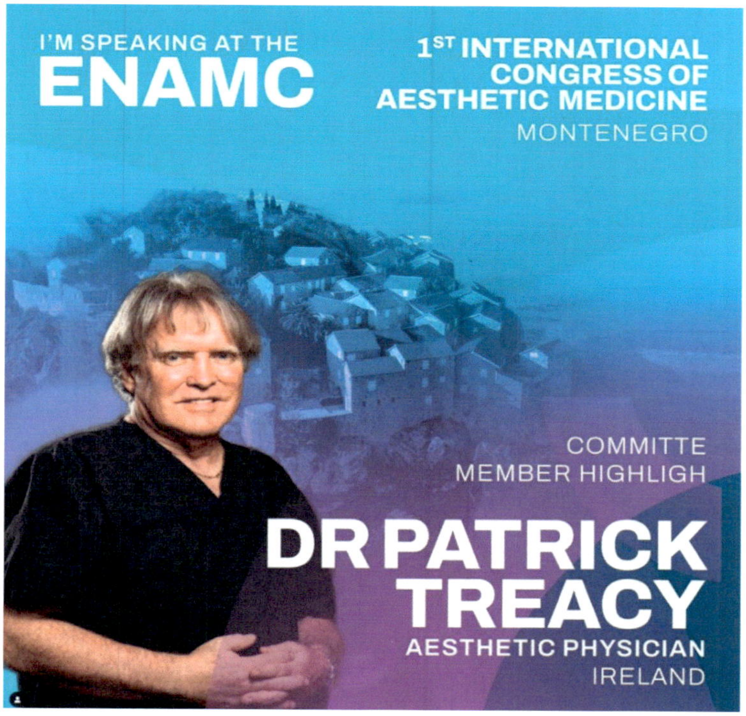

Beyond aesthetic applications, **growth factors** play a central role in **tissue engineering and regenerative medicine**, where they guide **stem cell differentiation** and stimulate **new tissue formation** in advanced therapies such as **bone grafts, cartilage repair, and skin substitutes**. Their influence extends to orchestrating complex regenerative processes, yet this same potency underscores a dual nature: while essential for normal healing and tissue maintenance, **dysregulated growth factor signaling** can inadvertently contribute to **tumour growth and angiogenesis**. This paradox has made them a focal point in **oncological research**, where targeted therapies—such as **VEGF inhibitors**—seek to counteract their pro-tumorigenic effects while preserving their regenerative benefits.

The **mechanism of action** of growth factors begins with their **binding to specific transmembrane receptors** on the surface of target cells, commonly **receptor tyrosine kinases (RTKs)** or **serine/threonine kinase receptors**. This **ligand–receptor interaction** triggers intracellular signaling cascades, most notably the **MAPK/ERK** and **PI3K/AKT** pathways, which modulate **gene expression, protein synthesis, and cellular behavior**. These pathways collectively drive outcomes such as **cell proliferation, differentiation, migration, and survival**, which are fundamental to tissue regeneration.

Importantly, **tight regulatory control**—through feedback loops, phosphatases, and inhibitory proteins—ensures that these signaling processes remain balanced. Without such regulation, overactivation can result in **uncontrolled cell proliferation** or **fibrosis**, while insufficient activation can impair healing.

Clinically, **growth factors are administered through various modalities**, including **localized injections**, **topical formulations**, and **biomaterial-based scaffolds** in tissue engineering. However, their **efficacy and safety** depend heavily on **precise dosing, targeted delivery, and controlled release kinetics**. Excessive or poorly localized exposure may lead to adverse effects such as **aberrant tissue growth**, **chronic inflammation**, or even **malignant transformation**. Consequently, ongoing research is focused on developing **smart delivery systems**—including **nanocarriers and exosome-based vectors**—to optimize therapeutic outcomes while minimizing risks.

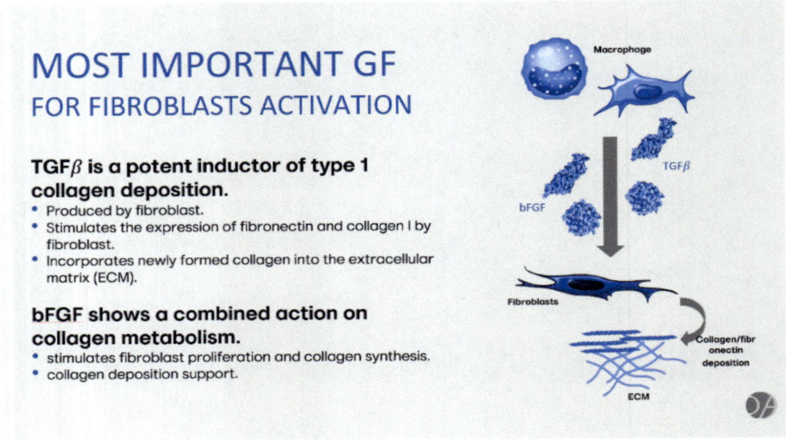

Advances in recombinant technology have revolutionized the large-scale production of **synthetic growth factors**, such as **epidermal growth factor (EGF)** for wound healing, significantly expanding their **therapeutic accessibility** and consistency. These innovations have made it possible to reproduce naturally occurring proteins with high purity and controlled potency, ensuring reliable outcomes across a range of clinical applications.

Despite their promise, the **clinical use of growth factors** demands **careful regulation and precision**. **Accurate dosing** and **tissue-specific delivery** are critical to achieving optimal safety and efficacy. Systemic or excessive administration can disrupt cellular signaling balance, leading to **unintended effects** such as **fibrosis**, **abnormal tissue proliferation**, or **increased malignancy risk**. Accordingly, **stringent regulatory oversight** and **well-designed clinical trials** are essential to validate their therapeutic profiles—particularly within **aesthetic medicine**, where patients expect both visible efficacy and uncompromised safety.

As research advances, **innovations in delivery systems**—including **controlled-release matrices**, **nanocarriers**, and **exosome-based formulations**—are enhancing the **precision, bioavailability, and localization** of growth factor therapies. Coupled with recombinant advancements, these technologies are paving the way for **next-generation regenerative treatments** that integrate biological intelligence with clinical control.

In **aesthetic medicine**, such progress promises **refined, minimally invasive approaches** to **skin rejuvenation**, **hair restoration**, and **tissue repair**, aligning with the growing demand for **biologically driven, restorative solutions**.

Ultimately, **growth factors represent foundational drivers of cellular regeneration**, offering transformative potential across **aesthetic and regenerative medicine**. Their capacity to **stimulate tissue repair**, **enhance skin and hair vitality**, and **support advanced therapeutic innovations** underscores their enduring clinical value. As precision-engineering techniques evolve, growth factor therapies will continue to **redefine the intersection of beauty and biology**, empowering clinicians to harness the body's innate regenerative power for safer, more natural results.

Q13 – Which Growth Factors are the most important in Aesthetic Medicine?

In the **rapidly advancing field of aesthetic medicine**, **growth factors** have emerged as **powerful biological allies**, harnessing the body's innate regenerative mechanisms to **rejuvenate skin**, **restore hair**, and **accelerate healing**. These **naturally occurring proteins and peptides** function as **key signaling molecules**, binding to **specific cellular receptors** to initiate cascades that drive **cell proliferation**, **differentiation**, and **extracellular matrix synthesis**.

Their remarkable **potency at low concentrations** allows them to produce profound biological effects, making them **indispensable tools** for enhancing **tissue repair**, **cellular renewal**, and **long-lasting aesthetic outcomes**. By stimulating **collagen production**, **angiogenesis**, and **cellular metabolism**, growth factors are **redefining modern aesthetics**—shifting the focus from superficial correction to **deep, regenerative rejuvenation**.

Through these mechanisms, clinicians can now offer patients **biologically intelligent treatments** that harmonize with the body's own healing capacity, reflecting the **core principles of regenerative medicine** and ushering in a new era of **science-driven beauty**.

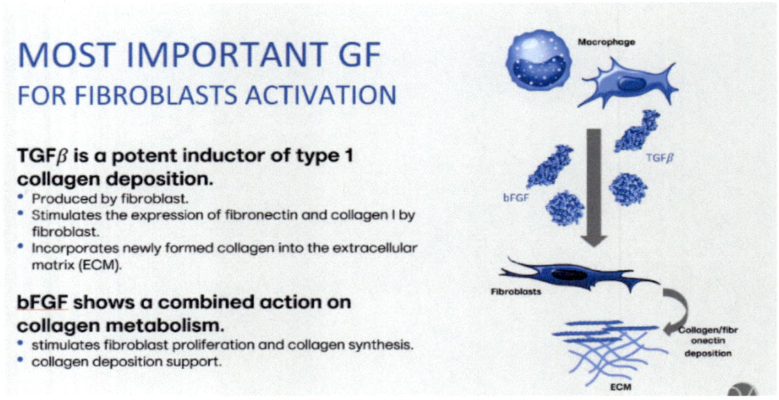

Among the most influential growth factors in aesthetic medicine is **Epidermal Growth Factor (EGF)**, which drives **cell proliferation and differentiation** within epithelial tissues, particularly the skin. EGF accelerates **wound healing**, enhances **post-procedural regeneration** following treatments such as **laser resurfacing** or **microneedling**, and improves overall **skin texture, tone, and radiance**, making it a **cornerstone of rejuvenation protocols**.

Fibroblast Growth Factors (FGFs) play a complementary role by promoting **angiogenesis** and stimulating the **synthesis of collagen and elastin**, key components that maintain **skin elasticity and structural integrity**. Similarly, **Platelet-Derived Growth Factor (PDGF)**—released during the clotting process—**recruits fibroblasts and smooth muscle cells** to sites of tissue injury, stimulating their proliferation and supporting **collagen formation**. This makes PDGF a critical mediator of **tissue repair and skin revitalization**, particularly in **platelet-rich plasma (PRP) therapies**.

Transforming Growth Factor Beta (TGF-β) regulates the delicate balance between **collagen synthesis and degradation**, preserving **skin firmness** and promoting **extracellular matrix homeostasis**. However, its activity must be carefully controlled, as excessive TGF-β signaling can lead to **fibrotic changes**—an important consideration in aesthetic applications.

Vascular Endothelial Growth Factor (VEGF) enhances aesthetic outcomes by stimulating **angiogenesis**, thereby improving **tissue oxygenation**, **nutrient delivery**, and **healing efficiency**. These effects are particularly beneficial in **skin rejuvenation** and **hair restoration** treatments. Meanwhile, **Insulin-Like Growth Factors (IGFs)** contribute to **tissue maintenance and repair**, reinforcing **skin vitality** and **hair follicle health** when used synergistically with other growth factors.

Connective Tissue Growth Factor (CTGF), often acting downstream of TGF-β, further promotes **collagen synthesis** and **extracellular matrix organization**. However, as with TGF-β, **overexpression** of CTGF has been linked to **fibrotic disorders**, emphasizing the importance of **precise regulatory control**.

Beyond these classical growth factors, **cytokines** such as **Interleukins (IL-1, IL-6)** play a vital supportive role by modulating **fibroblast activity** and **matrix remodeling**. They indirectly enhance tissue repair through **neovascularization**, often mediated by **VEGF**, improving **nutrient exchange** and **cellular waste clearance**, which together sustain **optimal skin regeneration**.

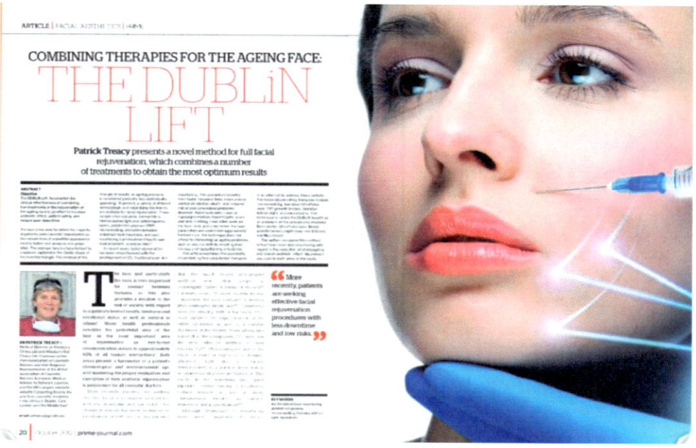
ARTICLE

COMBINING THERAPIES FOR THE AGEING FACE:

THE DUBLiN LIFT

Patrick Treacy presents a novel method for full facial rejuvenation, which combines a number of treatments to obtain the most optimum results

"More recently, patients are seeking effective facial rejuvenation procedures with less downtime and low risks"

The Dublin Lift technique was invented by Dr Patrick Treacy

The **clinical significance** of these growth factors lies in their **synergistic interactions**, which amplify their overall impact in aesthetic medicine. In **skin rejuvenation**, they stimulate **collagen and elastin synthesis**, reduce **fine lines and wrinkles**, and enhance **skin tone and texture**, achieving **natural, youthful results**. In **hair restoration**, growth factors revitalize **follicular activity**, improve **microvascular circulation** in the scalp, and support **robust, sustained hair growth**. Following aesthetic procedures, they accelerate **tissue recovery**, **reduce inflammation**, and **optimize healing**, thereby improving outcomes after treatments such as **laser resurfacing**, **chemical peels**, and **microneedling**.

These bioactive molecules are commonly delivered through **advanced therapeutic platforms**, including **platelet-rich plasma (PRP)**, **topical formulations**, and **exosome-based systems**, where their **combined regenerative effects** produce the most significant clinical benefits. The coordinated actions of **PDGF, TGF-β, FGFs, and EGF**—which collectively **chemoattract repair cells**, **stimulate proliferation**, and **enhance extracellular matrix production**—make them central to **tissue repair and remodeling**, reinforcing their widespread application in aesthetic protocols.

The **integration of growth factors** into aesthetic practice, however, demands **precise control and individualized planning** to maximize both **efficacy and safety**. Delivery through PRP, exosomes, or engineered biomaterials must be carefully **calibrated to target specific tissues**, as **excessive concentrations** or **systemic exposure** can potentially trigger **unintended effects**, such as **aberrant cell proliferation**.

Ongoing research continues to refine these therapies, investigating **optimal dosing**, **growth factor combinations**, and **delivery methods** to fully harness their regenerative potential. By deepening the understanding of how these molecules **interact within cellular networks**, clinicians can **personalize treatment strategies** to each patient's unique biology, achieving outcomes that elegantly blend **scientific precision with aesthetic artistry**.

As the field of aesthetic medicine evolves, the **strategic application of growth factors** is poised to **elevate standards of care**, offering patients **transformative, natural-looking results** rooted in the body's **intrinsic capacity for renewal and repair**.

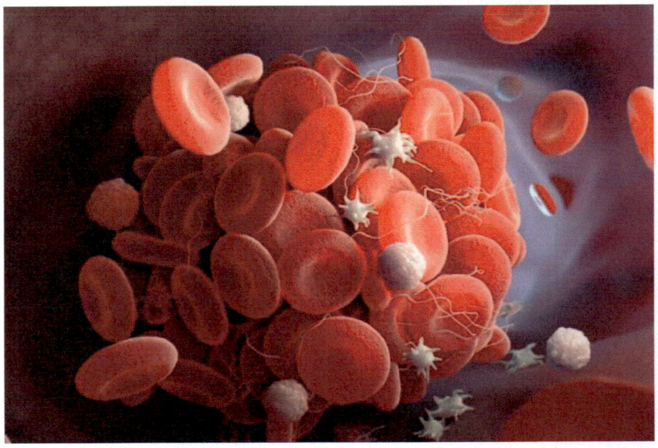

The **Dublin Lift** is a **composite aesthetic procedure**, its name often represented as an acronym (**DUBLiN**) reflecting its key components: **Dermaroller, Ultralase Laser, Blood-derived growth factors (PRP), Light therapy (near-red 633 nm),** and **Neurotoxin**. This innovative treatment is designed to **counteract skin aging** by **stimulating fibroblast activity**, thereby enhancing **collagen and elastin synthesis** and **promoting tissue regeneration and repair**.

Developed by **Dr. Patrick Treacy**, a recognized **pioneer in aesthetic medicine**, the Dublin Lift integrates multiple synergistic modalities to **leverage the body's innate regenerative mechanisms**. Its ability to **revitalize skin structure**, **improve tone and elasticity**, and **deliver natural, rejuvenated results** has earned it **international acclaim** as a benchmark in advanced aesthetic rejuvenation techniques.

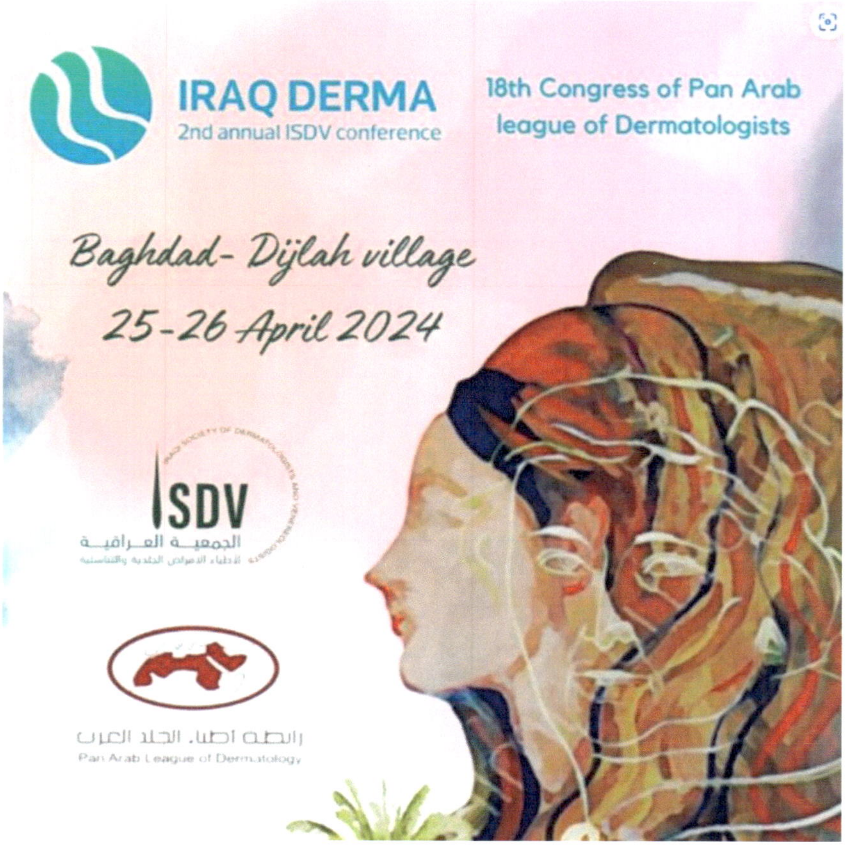

Dr Patrick Treacy spoke on the HELPIR technique at the 18th Congress of Pan Arab league of Dermatologists in Baghdad 2024

The **HELPIR Technique**—an acronym for **Hyaluronic Acid, Embryonic Stem Cells from Red Deer, Lasers, Platelet-Rich Plasma, Intense Pulsed Light,** and **Radiofrequency**—was a **multimodal aesthetic protocol** developed to **stimulate the body's intrinsic regenerative mechanisms** for comprehensive facial rejuvenation. By combining **red deer embryonic stem cells (ESCs)** with **PRP** and other regenerative modalities, the technique activated **biological pathways that enhance tissue repair, collagen synthesis, and cellular renewal**.

The inclusion of **red deer ESCs** represented a groundbreaking innovation, as **animal-derived stem cells** were seldom employed in aesthetic practice at the time Dr. Treacy introduced this method. These cells—presumably sourced from **early-stage embryonic or placental tissue**—exhibit a **high regenerative potential** owing to their **pluripotency** and secretion of **bioactive**

molecules, including **exosomes and growth factors**. This strategic choice marked a **notable departure from human-derived stem cell applications**, which are often constrained by **ethical and regulatory limitations**, positioning the HELPIR Technique as a **pioneering approach** in exploring **alternative, cross-species regenerative sources** within aesthetic medicine.

Q14 – What Is Platelet Rich Plasma and How Is It Prepared?

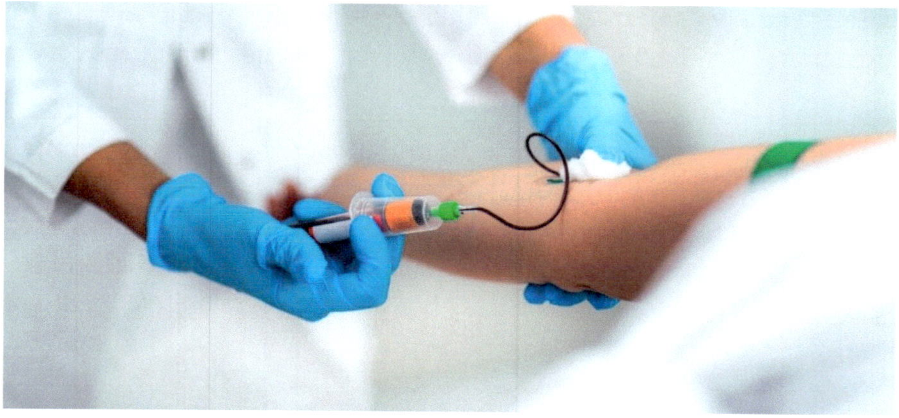

Platelet-Rich Plasma (PRP)—an autologous therapy derived from a patient's own blood—has become a cornerstone of aesthetic medicine, renowned for its capacity to **enhance tissue repair, stimulate collagen production, and rejuvenate both skin and hair**. By concentrating platelets and their associated growth factors, PRP delivers a **potent regenerative cocktail** that promotes natural, progressive improvements with minimal risk. In the hands of skilled practitioners, PRP has evolved far beyond a simple injectable; its integration into advanced protocols such as the **Dublin Lift** has elevated it into a **multifaceted rejuvenation strategy**, combining scientific precision with artistic application. The therapy exemplifies the **synergy of biology and aesthetics**, offering patients minimally invasive treatments that harness the body's intrinsic healing mechanisms for visible, enduring results.

The preparation of PRP begins with a **routine blood draw**, followed by **centrifugation** to separate the sample into distinct layers: red blood cells, platelet-poor plasma, and the coveted **platelet-rich fraction**. This PRP layer—dense with platelets and growth factors—is carefully extracted for therapeutic use. Once activated, the platelets release a **cascade of bioactive molecules**, including **Platelet-Derived Growth Factor (PDGF)**, **Transforming Growth Factor Beta (TGF-β)**, and **Vascular Endothelial Growth Factor (VEGF)**, alongside a variety of cytokines. These mediators orchestrate a complex regenerative process, stimulating **cell proliferation, collagen synthesis, angiogenesis, and tissue remodeling**. By promoting fibroblast division and extracellular matrix formation, PRP enhances **tissue strength, elasticity, and resilience**, while its angiogenic components encourage **new capillary growth** to support nutrient delivery and tissue vitality. Moreover, PRP's **anti-inflammatory and immunomodulatory properties** help regulate the healing response, minimizing scar formation and expediting recovery.

In aesthetic medicine, PRP's versatility makes it one of the most valuable tools in regenerative therapy. For **facial rejuvenation**, PRP may be **injected or applied topically** following microneedling to improve **skin texture, tone, and firmness**, while reducing **fine lines, wrinkles,**

and acne scars. In **hair restoration**, targeted scalp injections stimulate **dormant follicles**, increase **hair density**, and improve **scalp health**, offering a promising solution for certain forms of alopecia. PRP also plays a vital role in **scar revision**, particularly in the treatment of **acne or surgical scars**, where it accelerates healing and refines surface texture when used in combination with modalities such as **laser resurfacing** or **microneedling**. Post-procedure, PRP accelerates **tissue regeneration**, **reduces inflammation**, and **shortens downtime** after interventions like ablative laser treatments or chemical peels, thereby optimizing both recovery and aesthetic outcomes.

Because PRP is **autologous**—sourced directly from the patient—it carries **virtually no risk of allergic reaction or disease transmission**. Its **biocompatibility** and ability to **synergize with complementary treatments** make it an exceptionally adaptable component of modern aesthetic protocols. As the field continues to evolve, PRP remains a **foundational therapy in regenerative aesthetics**, bridging scientific innovation with the body's own regenerative intelligence.

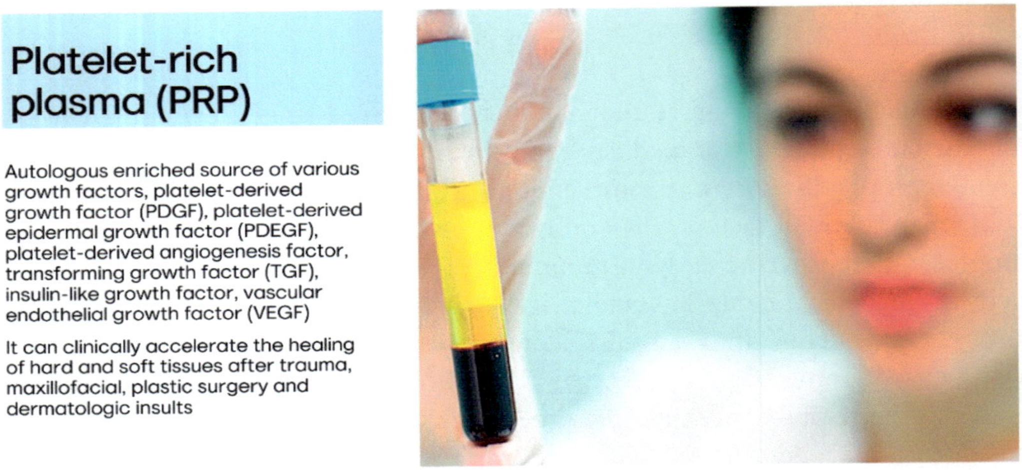

The efficacy of **Platelet-Rich Plasma (PRP)** therapy is highly **technique-sensitive**, with results dependent on variables such as **centrifugation protocols, platelet concentration, and injection techniques**. Patient-related factors—including **overall health, nutritional status, and platelet functionality**—also significantly influence therapeutic outcomes. Because PRP stimulates gradual biological regeneration, its benefits are typically **cumulative**, often requiring a **series of sessions spaced over several weeks or months** to achieve optimal and sustained results. **Regulatory compliance** is equally essential, as practitioners must adhere to local and international guidelines governing PRP preparation, handling, and clinical application to ensure both safety and efficacy.

Despite these technical and procedural considerations, PRP's **minimal downtime**, **autologous nature**, and **biological compatibility** make it an appealing choice for patients seeking **natural, minimally invasive regenerative treatments**. Its transformative potential is perhaps best demonstrated in **Dr. Patrick Treacy's multi-award-winning Dublin Lift**, a pioneering **combi-procedural protocol** designed for facial rejuvenation and adaptable for hair restoration. Within the Dublin Lift, PRP serves as a **central regenerative component**, leveraging its **growth factor–**

rich and **cell-stimulating properties** to enhance **collagen synthesis, promote tissue repair**, and achieve **subtle yet long-lasting improvements** in both skin and hair quality.

The **Dublin Lift** exemplifies how PRP can be **integrated into a sophisticated, multi-modal aesthetic strategy**. By combining PRP with complementary modalities—such as **laser treatments, dermal stimulation, and light-based therapies**—the protocol amplifies regenerative outcomes by targeting the **cellular and molecular mechanisms** underlying rejuvenation. The growth factors released from PRP, including **Platelet-Derived Growth Factor (PDGF)**, **Transforming Growth Factor Beta (TGF-β)**, and **Vascular Endothelial Growth Factor (VEGF)**, act synergistically to **recruit immune cells, fibroblasts, and stem cells** to the treated area. This orchestrated response initiates **early tissue repair**, **stimulates cellular proliferation**, and **remodels collagen fibers**, resulting in improved **tissue strength, elasticity, and hydration**.

This **balanced regenerative cascade** not only enhances aesthetic outcomes but also supports **rapid recovery with minimal scarring**, aligning with the Dublin Lift's philosophy of delivering **refined, natural-looking transformations**. As ongoing research continues to optimize **PRP formulation, concentration, and delivery techniques**, its role in aesthetic medicine—**exemplified by the innovation and success of the Dublin Lift**—is poised to expand further. Together, these advancements affirm PRP's place as a **cornerstone of regenerative aesthetics**, offering patients a powerful, biologically driven pathway to renewed beauty and vitality.

Q15 – What Is Platelet Rich Fibrin and How Is It Prepared?

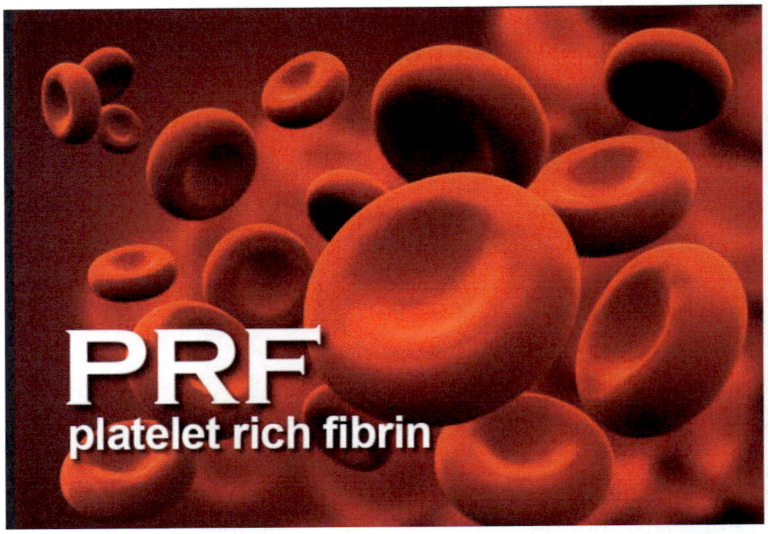

Platelet-Rich Fibrin (PRF)—a second-generation platelet concentrate derived from a patient's own blood—represents a major advancement in regenerative and aesthetic medicine, offering a **natural, additive-free** approach to tissue repair and rejuvenation. Unlike **Platelet-Rich Plasma (PRP)**, which remains in liquid form and often requires the use of anticoagulants, PRF forms a **gel-like fibrin matrix** that entraps **platelets, leukocytes, and growth factors**, enabling a **gradual and sustained release** of regenerative signals over time. This unique **three-dimensional fibrin scaffold**, enriched with **Platelet-Derived Growth Factor (PDGF)**, **Transforming Growth Factor Beta (TGF-β)**, and **Vascular Endothelial Growth Factor (VEGF)**, provides structural integrity while supporting prolonged cellular activity and tissue regeneration. Through this mechanism, PRF enhances **cell migration, angiogenesis, and collagen synthesis**, making it a powerful, biocompatible tool for **skin rejuvenation, wound healing, and tissue repair**. By leveraging the body's intrinsic healing mechanisms, PRF aligns perfectly with the modern shift toward **biologically driven, minimally invasive aesthetic treatments**.

The preparation of PRF is **simple yet highly technique-sensitive**, requiring both precision and timing. The process begins with a **small venous blood draw**, typically between **10 and 20 millilitres**, collected into **specialized glass or anticoagulant-free tubes**. Immediate centrifugation—usually within **one to two minutes of collection** to prevent premature clotting—is critical. The sample is spun at a **controlled speed and duration**, commonly around **2700 rpm for 8–12 minutes**, depending on the selected protocol. This centrifugation separates the blood components by density: **red blood cells** settle at the bottom, **platelet-poor plasma** forms a clear layer at the top, and the **fibrin clot**, or **"buffy coat,"** rich in platelets, leukocytes, and growth factors, develops in the middle.

Because PRF is produced without anticoagulants, the blood undergoes **natural coagulation**, forming a **dense fibrin network** that entraps regenerative elements within its matrix. This fibrin structure acts as a **biological reservoir**, gradually releasing growth factors and cytokines over several days, sustaining cellular stimulation and healing responses. Once formed, the **PRF clot** is carefully extracted under sterile conditions, and any residual red blood cells are gently removed to yield a **pliable, amber-colored fibrin membrane** suitable for clinical application. This membrane can be **used immediately**, either **placed directly into treatment sites**—such as dermal planes, surgical wounds, or scalp tissues—or **combined with complementary aesthetic procedures** like microneedling, laser therapy, or filler injections to amplify regenerative outcomes.

Q16 – Tell me about the Award-Winning DUBLIN Lift

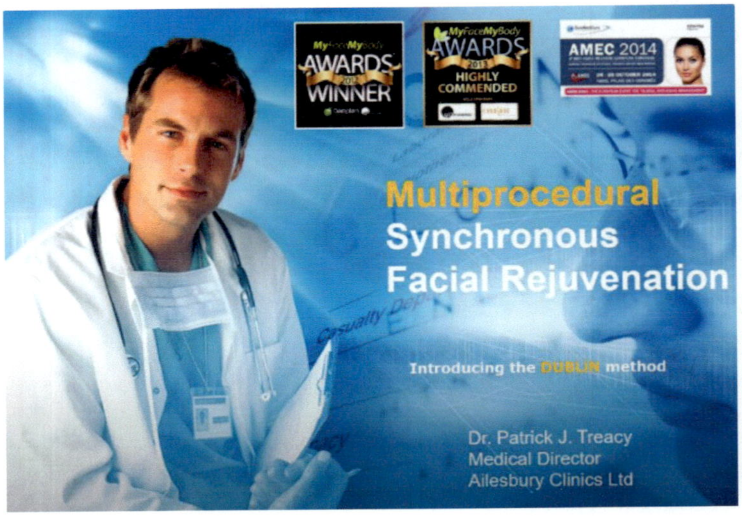

The Dublin Lift, a **multi-award-winning combiprocedural protocol** developed by **Dr. Patrick Treacy**, has redefined both **facial and hair rejuvenation** by harnessing the body's innate regenerative potential through a **synergistic fusion of advanced therapies**. Recognized internationally with the **MyFaceMyBody Award (London, 2012)** and the **AMEC Award (Paris, 2014)**, this pioneering approach originally combined **Platelet-Rich Plasma (PRP)**, **microneedling**, and **near-red light therapy (633 nm)** to deliver natural, biologically driven rejuvenation. The protocol later evolved into the **Dublin Lift PLUS**, incorporating **mesenchymal stem cells** to further amplify tissue repair and regeneration.

Represented by the acronym **DUBLiN—Dermaroller (microneedling), Umbilical stem cells, Blood growth factors (PRP), Light (near-red 633 nm)**, and **Neurotoxin**—the Dublin Lift seamlessly integrates these elements to achieve **long-lasting aesthetic improvements with minimal downtime**. By leveraging the synergistic action of **growth factors, cytokines, and stem cell–derived signaling molecules**, this holistic technique addresses multiple dimensions of aging. Patients experience **smoother skin texture**, **reduced fine lines and wrinkles**, and **enhanced hair density**, all achieved through a **regenerative, rather than purely corrective, approach** to aesthetics.

At the heart of the Dublin Lift lies **microneedling**, which employs precision instruments such as the **Dermaroller** to create **controlled micro-injuries** within the epidermis and dermis. These microscopic punctures **activate the skin's wound-healing cascade**, stimulating **fibroblast activity**, **collagen and elastin synthesis**, and **accelerated cellular turnover**. Crucially, microneedling also generates **microchannels** that enhance the transdermal absorption and efficacy of regenerative agents like **PRP** or **stem cell concentrates**.

PRP, derived from a patient's own blood through centrifugation, is rich in **Platelet-Derived Growth Factor (PDGF)**, **Transforming Growth Factor Beta (TGF-β)**, and **Vascular Endothelial Growth Factor (VEGF)**. When applied to microneedled skin or injected into target areas such as the **face or scalp**, these growth factors **stimulate fibroblast proliferation**, **promote angiogenesis**, **accelerate collagen remodeling**, and **revitalize cellular metabolism**. The result is **improved skin elasticity**, **diminished wrinkles and scars**, and **reactivated hair follicles**, leading to visibly denser and healthier hair.

Complementing these effects, **near-red light therapy at 633 nm** enhances **mitochondrial activity** and **upregulates collagen gene expression**, thereby accelerating **tissue repair** and **reducing post-treatment recovery time**. Together, these modalities form a comprehensive, biologically synergistic system that epitomizes the future of regenerative aesthetics—**restoring youthfulness not by masking age, but by revitalizing the body's own healing intelligence**.

At the core of the **Dublin Lift** lies **microneedling**, which employs devices ranging from the **classic Dermaroller** to more advanced systems such as the **Dermapen** and **SkinPen** to create **controlled micro-injuries** within the epidermis and dermis. These precisely calibrated microchannels **activate the skin's natural wound-healing cascade**, stimulating **fibroblast activity**, **collagen and elastin synthesis**, and **accelerated cellular turnover**. In addition to triggering regeneration, the microchannels enhance the **transdermal absorption** of bioactive agents, improving the efficacy of **Platelet-Rich Plasma (PRP)** and **stem cell–based concentrates**.

PRP, prepared through centrifugation of a patient's own blood to concentrate platelets and their associated growth factors—including **Platelet-Derived Growth Factor (PDGF)**, **Transforming Growth Factor Beta (TGF-β)**, and **Vascular Endothelial Growth Factor (VEGF)**—is applied either **topically over microneedled skin** or **injected into targeted areas** such as the **face** or **scalp**. These potent biomolecules **stimulate fibroblast proliferation**, **promote collagen synthesis**, **induce angiogenesis**, and **revitalize cellular metabolism**, collectively improving skin texture, elasticity, and tone. The outcome is a visible reduction in **fine lines, wrinkles, and scarring**, as well as the **reactivation of dormant hair follicles**, resulting in enhanced hair density and scalp vitality.

Near-red light therapy (633 nm) further augments these regenerative effects by **stimulating mitochondrial activity**, enhancing **adenosine triphosphate (ATP) production**, and **upregulating collagen gene expression**. This photobiomodulation accelerates **tissue repair**, reduces **inflammation**, and minimizes **post-procedure downtime**, allowing faster recovery and improved treatment outcomes. In **2017**, the protocol was further refined to include **Microneedling Radiofrequency (MNRF)**, which combines the collagen-inducing benefits of microneedling with the **thermal stimulation of radiofrequency energy**, yielding deeper dermal remodeling and enhanced skin tightening.

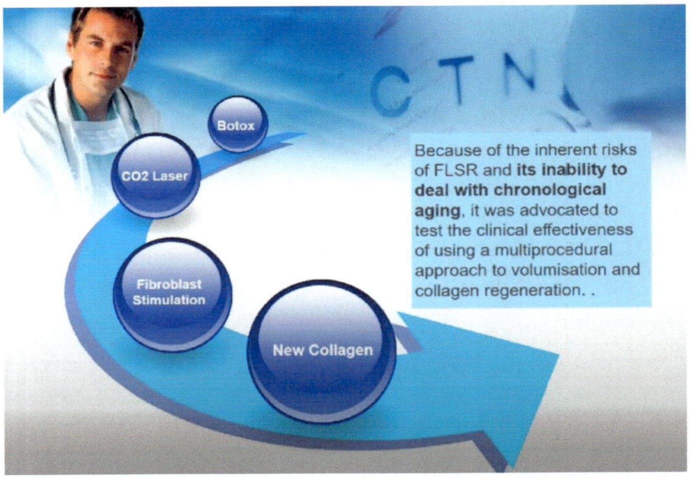

The introduction of **mesenchymal stem cells (MSCs)**—sourced from **umbilical cord** or **adipose tissue**—marked a major advancement in the evolution of the **Dublin Lift PLUS** technique. These pluripotent cells possess **self-renewal capacity** and the ability to **differentiate into multiple cellular lineages**, while secreting a **bioactive secretome** rich in **growth factors**, **cytokines**, and **extracellular vesicles**, including **exosomes**. This molecular cocktail amplifies **angiogenesis**, **collagen remodeling**, and **tissue regeneration**, substantially enhancing the treatment's restorative power—particularly for patients seeking **comprehensive rejuvenation** or those with more advanced signs of aging.

To complement these regenerative modalities, **Botulinum Toxin Type A (neurotoxin)** is integrated into the protocol to **relax dynamic facial muscles**, thereby **smoothing expression lines** and **refining surface texture**. This strategic addition not only enhances aesthetic harmony but also prolongs the youthful, polished results achieved through the regenerative actions of **microneedling, PRP, and MSC therapy**.

Together, these synergistic components form a **comprehensive, biologically driven rejuvenation system** that targets the manifestations of aging at both the **cellular** and **structural** levels—restoring vitality, resilience, and balance to the skin and hair through the body's own regenerative intelligence.

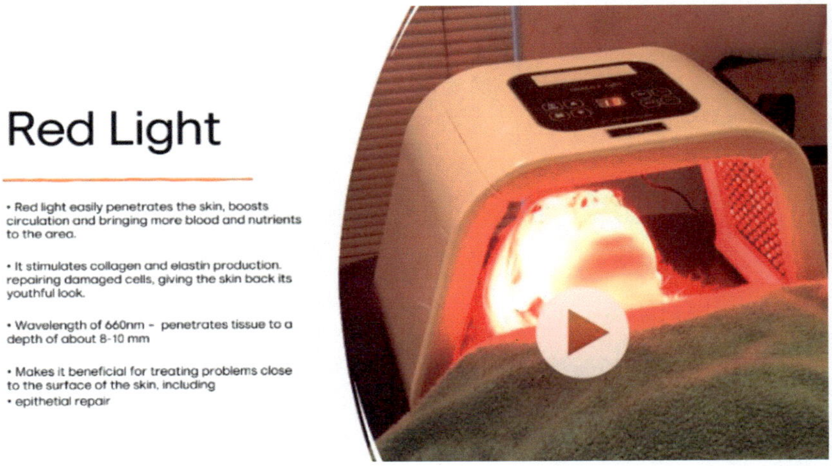

The success of the **Dublin Lift** lies in the **synergistic interplay of growth factors and cytokines**, which coordinate cellular communication and regeneration at multiple biological levels. Key growth factors—**Platelet-Derived Growth Factor (PDGF)**, **Transforming Growth Factor Beta (TGF-β)**, and **Fibroblast Growth Factor (FGF)**—bind to fibroblast receptors to stimulate **collagen and elastin synthesis**, reinforcing the skin's structural integrity. Meanwhile, **Vascular Endothelial Growth Factor (VEGF)** and FGF drive **angiogenesis**, improving microcirculation and facilitating the **delivery of oxygen and nutrients** while promoting the **removal of metabolic waste** from treated tissues. This enhanced vascular support accelerates tissue repair, improves dermal vitality, and optimizes **hair follicle function** in restoration procedures.

Cytokines, including anti-inflammatory mediators, finely regulate the healing environment by **modulating inflammation** to prevent excessive tissue response and ensure smooth recovery. Concurrently, **matrix metalloproteinases (MMPs)**—enzymes modulated by cytokines—break down damaged components of the **extracellular matrix (ECM)**, creating space for **new collagen deposition** and **organized tissue remodeling** under the influence of growth factors. The inclusion of **stem cell secretomes** further enhances this process through **bioactive signaling molecules**, **exosomes**, and **cytokines** that reduce inflammation, promote **neovascularization**, and activate resident **fibroblasts** and **keratinocytes**, thereby amplifying the regenerative cascade and extending the therapeutic benefits.

Clinical outcomes of the Dublin Lift, evaluated using standardized measures such as the **Wrinkle Severity Rating Scale (WSRS)** and the **Global Aesthetic Improvement Scale (GAIS)**, demonstrate significant improvements in **skin texture**, **wrinkle depth**, and overall **dermal rejuvenation**. Patients consistently report **smoother, firmer skin**, and, in the context of **hair restoration**, increased **density** and a **fuller appearance**. These outcomes are supported by **photographic documentation** and high **patient satisfaction scores**, underscoring the reproducibility and efficacy of the technique.

The Dublin Lift distinguishes itself as a **comprehensive, minimally invasive rejuvenation protocol** that integrates **collagen induction**, **growth factor enrichment**, **cellular metabolic stimulation**, and **targeted neuromodulation** to deliver **natural, progressive improvements** without the stiffness or overcorrection often associated with traditional procedures. Its **international recognition** through accolades such as the **MyFaceMyBody Award (London, 2012)** and **AMEC Award (Paris, 2014)** attests to its innovation and clinical relevance. Moreover, its **evolution into the Dublin Lift PLUS technique**—incorporating **mesenchymal stem cell therapies**—reflects **Dr. Patrick Treacy's** ongoing commitment to advancing regenerative aesthetics and redefining the future of **biologically based rejuvenation**.

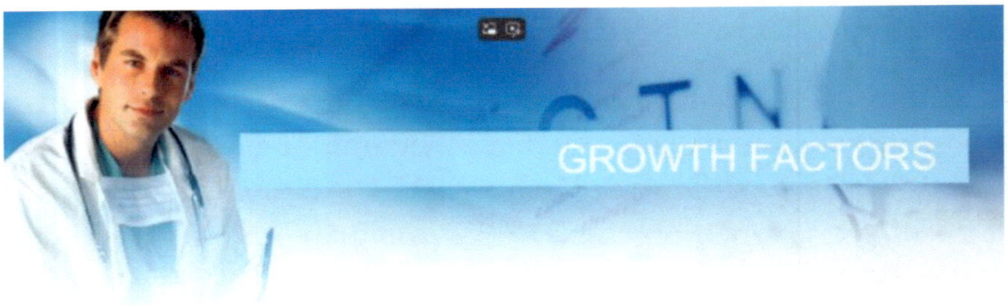

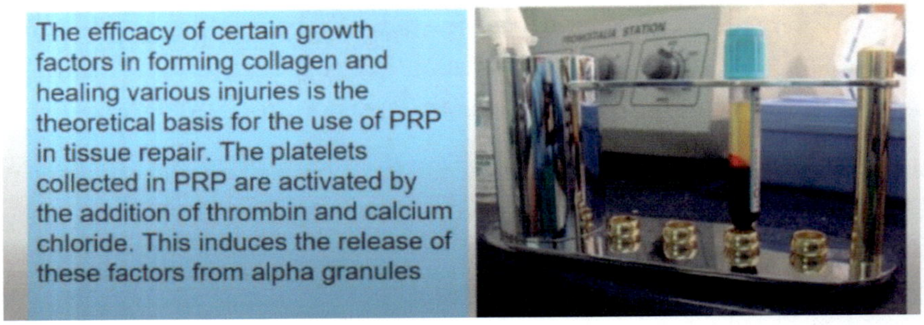

The **Dublin Lift** stands as a **pinnacle of innovation in aesthetic medicine**, earning international recognition through prestigious honors such as the **MyFaceMyBody Award (2012)** and the **AMEC Award (2014)**. This **multi-award-winning combiprocedural protocol** distinguishes itself with a **comprehensive, synergistic approach** that targets multiple dimensions of aging simultaneously, achieving **natural, long-lasting rejuvenation** for both **facial** and **hair restoration** applications.

By integrating **microneedling** for **collagen induction**, **Platelet-Rich Plasma (PRP)** for **growth factor enrichment**, **near-red light therapy (633 nm)** for **cellular metabolic enhancement**, **mesenchymal stem cells** for **amplified tissue regeneration**, and **Botulinum Toxin A** for **dynamic wrinkle relaxation**, the Dublin Lift—represented by the acronym **DUBLiN** (*Dermaroller, Umbilical stem cells, Blood growth factors, Light, Neurotoxin*)—offers a **holistic, biologically driven solution** that redefines aesthetic care. Its evolution into the **PLUS technique**, incorporating mesenchymal stem cells, exemplifies **Dr. Patrick Treacy's commitment** to pioneering **regenerative strategies**, ensuring the protocol's continued leadership and clinical relevance as of **June 2025**.

What sets the Dublin Lift apart is its **strategic fusion of minimally invasive techniques** that maximize **collagen remodeling**, **cellular renewal**, and **tissue repair**—all while minimizing downtime. **Microneedling** induces controlled micro-injuries to activate **fibroblast proliferation** and **collagen synthesis**, while **PRP** delivers a concentrated source of **growth factors** such as **PDGF**, **TGF-β**, and **VEGF**, which promote **angiogenesis** and enhance **dermal structure**. **Near-red light therapy** at 633 nm stimulates **mitochondrial function** and **cellular energy production**, accelerating healing and optimizing results. The addition of **mesenchymal stem cells**, sourced from **umbilical cord** or **adipose tissue**, introduces a **potent secretome** rich in **exosomes**, **cytokines**, and **bioactive growth factors**, further amplifying regenerative outcomes. Finally,

Botulinum Toxin A smooths **dynamic facial lines**, complementing the regenerative effects to create a **refined, youthful appearance**.

This **synergistic integration** of advanced modalities ensures **gradual, natural results** that harmonize with the body's intrinsic healing mechanisms—delivering rejuvenation that is both **scientifically grounded** and **aesthetically authentic**, without the artificiality often associated with conventional cosmetic interventions.

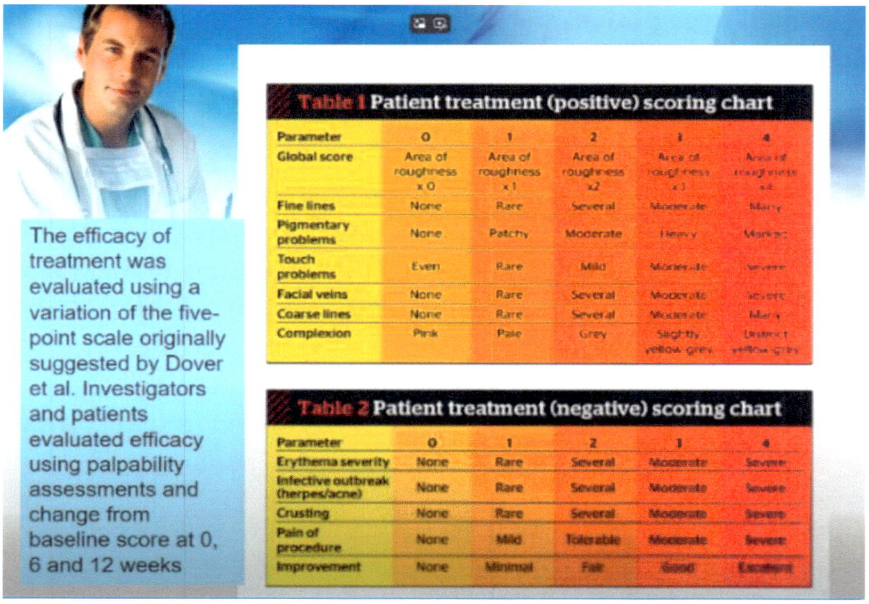

Table 1 Patient treatment (positive) scoring chart

Parameter	0	1	2	3	4
Global score	Area of roughness x 0	Area of roughness x 1	Area of roughness x2	Area of roughness x3	Area of roughness x4
Fine lines	None	Rare	Several	Moderate	Many
Pigmentary problems	None	Patchy	Moderate	Heavy	Marked
Touch problems	Even	Rare	Mild	Moderate	Severe
Facial veins	None	Rare	Several	Moderate	Severe
Coarse lines	None	Rare	Several	Moderate	Many
Complexion	Pink	Pale	Grey	Slightly yellow-grey	Distinct yellow-grey

Table 2 Patient treatment (negative) scoring chart

Parameter	0	1	2	3	4
Erythema severity	None	Rare	Several	Moderate	Severe
Infective outbreak (herpes/acne)	None	Rare	Several	Moderate	Severe
Crusting	None	Rare	Several	Moderate	Severe
Pain of procedure	None	Mild	Tolerable	Moderate	Severe
Improvement	None	Minimal	Fair	Good	Excellent

The **biological efficacy** of the **Dublin Lift** is driven by the **orchestrated interplay of growth factors and cytokines**, which form the foundation of its regenerative success. **Growth factors** such as **Platelet-Derived Growth Factor (PDGF)**, **Transforming Growth Factor Beta (TGF-β)**, and **Vascular Endothelial Growth Factor (VEGF)** directly stimulate **fibroblast activity**, promoting **collagen synthesis** and **extracellular matrix organization** to enhance **tissue strength, elasticity, and firmness** while reducing **wrinkles, scarring, and skin laxity**. **Cytokines** serve as key mediators of **cellular communication**, orchestrating the recruitment of **immune cells**, modulating **inflammatory responses**, and guiding **reparative cells** such as **fibroblasts** and **stem cells** toward tissue regeneration. **Matrix metalloproteinases (MMPs)**, regulated by cytokines, facilitate the **remodeling of damaged matrix components**, creating the structural framework for new collagen deposition under the direction of growth factors.

The **stem cell secretome**, rich in **bioactive molecules** such as **microRNAs**, **growth factors**, and **cytokines**, further amplifies this regenerative process by **reducing inflammation**, **enhancing vascularization**, and **stimulating resident cells** like **fibroblasts** and **keratinocytes**. This intricate cascade establishes a **powerful biological feedback loop** that drives the **Dublin Lift's transformative rejuvenation outcomes**.

The protocol's **minimal downtime** and **natural progression of results** make it especially appealing to patients seeking **effective yet subtle aesthetic enhancement**. By harnessing the body's own **innate regenerative mechanisms**, the Dublin Lift delivers **gradual, harmonious improvements** that align with the **natural rhythm of tissue renewal**. Clinical evaluations using the **Wrinkle Severity Rating Scale (WSRS)** and **Global Aesthetic Improvement Scale (GAIS)** consistently demonstrate **significant reductions in wrinkle depth**, **improved skin texture**, and **increased hair density** in restoration cases—findings further validated by **patient satisfaction surveys** and **photographic evidence**.

The procedure's **global recognition** underscores its **innovative and evidence-based nature**, while its **ongoing evolution** through the **PLUS technique**, incorporating **advanced stem cell therapies**, reflects **Dr. Patrick Treacy's dedication** to continually advancing the frontiers of **regenerative aesthetics**.

The **Dublin Lift's success** ultimately lies in its ability to **harness the synergy** of biologically active components—**growth factors, cytokines, and the stem cell secretome**—within a framework of **clinically validated therapies** such as **microneedling, platelet-rich plasma (PRP), and near-red light**, further enhanced by **targeted neurotoxin use**. This **holistic, multimodal approach** not only reverses visible signs of aging but also strengthens tissue health at a biological level, providing both **immediate and long-term rejuvenation**. The technique continues to **set a benchmark for excellence** in aesthetic medicine, offering patients a **transformative yet natural pathway to renewal** that balances innovation with biological harmony.

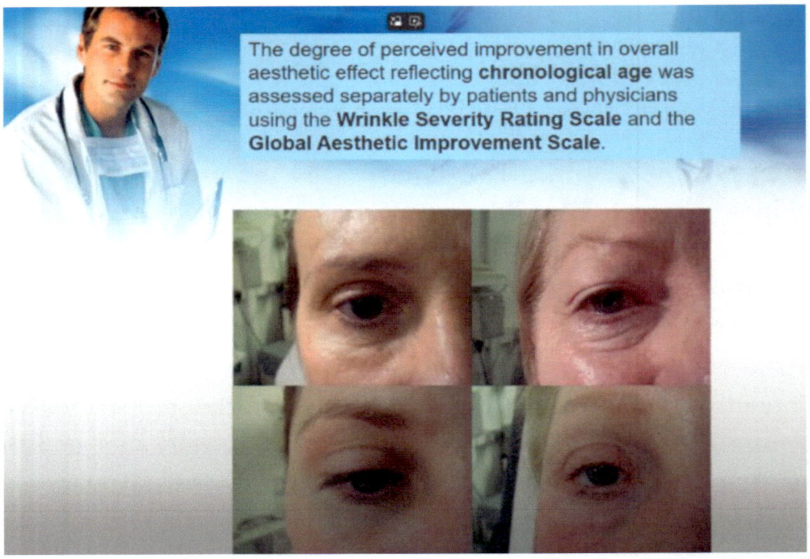

At its inception, the **Dublin Lift** combined **microneedling** to trigger collagen synthesis, **PRP** to deliver regenerative growth factors such as **PDGF**, **TGF-β**, and **VEGF**, and **near-red light therapy** to enhance cellular metabolism—creating a synergistic foundation for **tissue repair and renewal**. The incorporation of **Botulinum Toxin A** added a smoothing effect on **dynamic wrinkles**, complementing the regenerative elements. However, the introduction of **mesenchymal**

stem cell (MSC)–derived therapies, particularly through **Calecim Professional Serum**, marked a **pivotal evolution** in the protocol's regenerative power.

Dr. Treacy identified **Calecim's potent blend** of MSC-derived **growth factors** and **exosomes** as a breakthrough, even in its early formulations originally designed for general skin rejuvenation. Derived from **umbilical cord lining mesenchymal stem cells**, Calecim's **conditioned media** contained a rich "soup" of **bioactive molecules**—including **growth factors, cytokines, proteins, and exosomes**—that supported **cellular renewal**, **reduced inflammation**, and **enhanced tissue repair**. By 2012, Dr. Treacy was among the **first internationally** to integrate this serum at the **Ailesbury Clinic**, applying it for **hair follicle stimulation** and **skin rejuvenation** with remarkable outcomes that would later define a new paradigm in **regenerative aesthetics**.

The **scientific significance** of **Calecim Professional Serum** lies in its **exosome-rich composition**, reflecting the **paracrine activity** of MSCs. **Exosomes**, nano-sized extracellular vesicles (30–150 nm), transport **proteins, mRNAs, microRNAs, and lipids**, enabling **precise intercellular communication** and modulation of **cellular behavior**. Within the **Dublin Lift**, exosomes delivered through **microneedling** or **derma stamping** enhanced **fibroblast proliferation**, **collagen synthesis**, and **angiogenesis**, while reducing **inflammation** by up to **30-fold**, as supported by Calecim's clinical data.

This **cell-free approach** offered significant advantages over direct **MSC transplantation**, which can carry risks such as **immune rejection**, **tumorigenicity**, and **vascular occlusion**. By using **MSC-derived exosomes**, the technique avoided these complications while amplifying **regenerative efficacy**, demonstrating a **safer and more scalable model** for tissue restoration. Dr. Treacy's early adoption of this technology in 2012 **anticipated the global shift** toward **exosome-based therapeutics**, now gaining momentum across fields including **orthopedics**, **neurology**, and **oncology**.

The **Dublin Lift's pioneering integration** of **exosome-rich Calecim serum** foreshadowed broader applications in **regenerative medicine**, where **MSC-derived exosomes** are now recognized for their **immunomodulatory** and **tissue-repairing properties**. Research from **2018 to 2023** demonstrates exosomes' ability to **restore cartilage in osteoarthritis**, **accelerate wound healing**, and **modulate inflammation** in conditions such as **Alzheimer's disease** and **acute respiratory distress syndrome (ARDS)**. In aesthetics, exosomes from **MSCs** and **induced pluripotent stem cells (iPSCs)** have been shown to **reduce cellular senescence**, **stimulate collagen production**, and **enhance skin elasticity**, aligning closely with the Dublin Lift's clinical outcomes of **firmer, smoother skin** and **denser hair regrowth**.

The **integration of Calecim's PTT-6 formulation**, a patented blend of **MSC-derived growth factors and exosomes**, within the **Dublin Lift PLUS protocol**, further optimized delivery to **hair follicles** and **skin tissue**, producing **consistent and accelerated results** for conditions such as **telogen effluvium**, **postpartum hair loss**, and **early-stage androgenetic alopecia**. Patient feedback from the **Ailesbury Clinic** consistently reported **reduced scalp visibility**, **improved density**, and even **restoration of natural pigment**, underscoring the **protocol's transformative impact**.

Beyond its clinical achievements, the **Dublin Lift** has served as a **conceptual blueprint** for **next-generation regenerative therapies**. Its **synergistic framework**—combining **microneedling-induced micro-injury**, **PRP-mediated growth factor delivery**, **near-red light–driven metabolic enhancement**, and **exosome-based cellular signaling**—demonstrated how **multiple biological pathways** could be leveraged in concert for enhanced outcomes. This integrative model has since inspired applications such as **biomaterial-assisted exosome delivery** in orthopedics and **targeted exosome therapy** for neurological repair, capitalizing on exosomes' capacity to **cross the blood–brain barrier**.

The **Dublin Lift's minimal downtime**, **natural-appearing results**, and **biologically driven repair mechanisms** established a **new patient-centered standard** in regenerative aesthetics—prioritizing **safety, efficacy, and ethical sourcing**. Dr. Treacy's **early foresight** in utilizing Calecim serum long before **exosomes became mainstream in skincare** positioned the technique as a **visionary protocol** bridging **aesthetic innovation** and **biomedical science**.

Despite its pioneering status, the field remains subject to **regulatory complexities**. As of **June 2025**, the **U.S. FDA** confirms that **no exosome-based products** are currently approved for specific therapeutic or aesthetic use, citing concerns regarding **safety, efficacy, and unsubstantiated claims**. The **Dublin Lift**, however, has maintained its reputation through the **ethical integration** of **Calecim serum**, supported by **peer-reviewed clinical research** and **responsible sourcing** from **umbilical cord MSCs**.

Its outcomes—validated through **objective scales** such as the **Wrinkle Severity Rating Scale (WSRS)** and **Global Aesthetic Improvement Scale (GAIS)**, as well as high **patient satisfaction rates**—reinforce the protocol's **scientific credibility and safety profile**. By paving the way for **exosome-centered regenerative therapies**, the **Dublin Lift PLUS protocol** has not only **redefined aesthetic rejuvenation** but also **catalyzed progress across regenerative medicine**, leaving a lasting legacy of **biologically intelligent, ethically grounded innovation**.

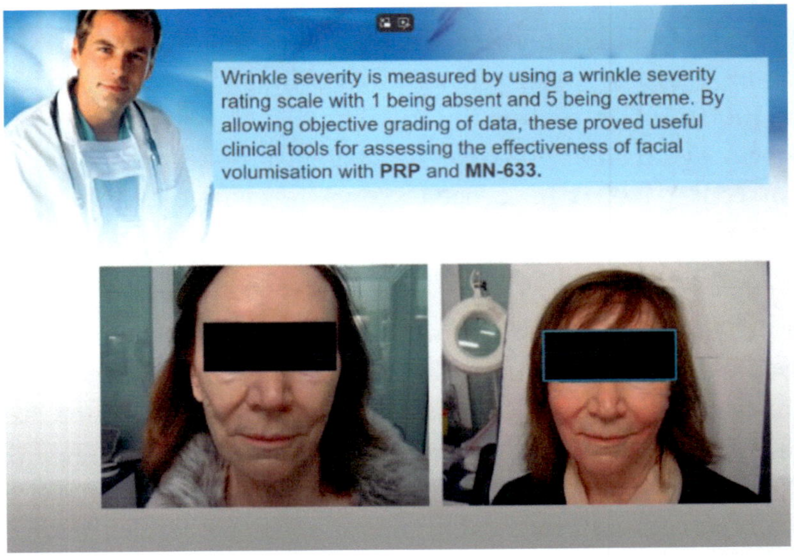

The **Wrinkle Severity Rating Scale (WSRS)** is a **standardized and validated clinical tool** used to quantify the **severity of facial wrinkles**, particularly **nasolabial folds**, in aesthetic and dermatologic practice. It offers a **consistent and reproducible method** for assessing **wrinkle depth and volume loss**, facilitating **treatment planning**, **outcome monitoring**, and **comparative analysis** across clinical studies. Originally developed for evaluating responses to **dermal fillers** and other **anti-aging interventions**, the WSRS is now **widely recognized** in both **dermatology** and **cosmetic surgery** as a benchmark measure of facial rejuvenation outcomes.

Structure and Scoring

The WSRS employs a **five-point ordinal scale**, with grades assigned based on **visual and tactile evaluation** of wrinkle depth and skin laxity:

- **Grade 1 (Absent):** No visible fold; the skin surface appears smooth and continuous.
- **Grade 2 (Mild):** A shallow yet visible fold with slight indentation; minimal disruption of skin texture.
- **Grade 3 (Moderate):** A moderately deep fold visible at rest, approximately 1–2 mm in depth; mild skin laxity may be present.
- **Grade 4 (Severe):** A deep, well-defined fold visible at rest, 2–4 mm in depth, accompanied by noticeable skin laxity.
- **Grade 5 (Very Severe):** A very deep fold with redundant skin and marked volume loss; depth exceeds 4 mm.

Assessments are typically performed by a **trained clinician** under **controlled lighting** and **neutral facial positioning**, ensuring standardized conditions. Evaluations may be conducted **at rest or during facial animation**, depending on the treatment focus. While the WSRS was primarily validated for **nasolabial folds**, it can be **adapted** for use on other facial regions—such as the **forehead, perioral, or periorbital areas**—with appropriate clinical judgment.

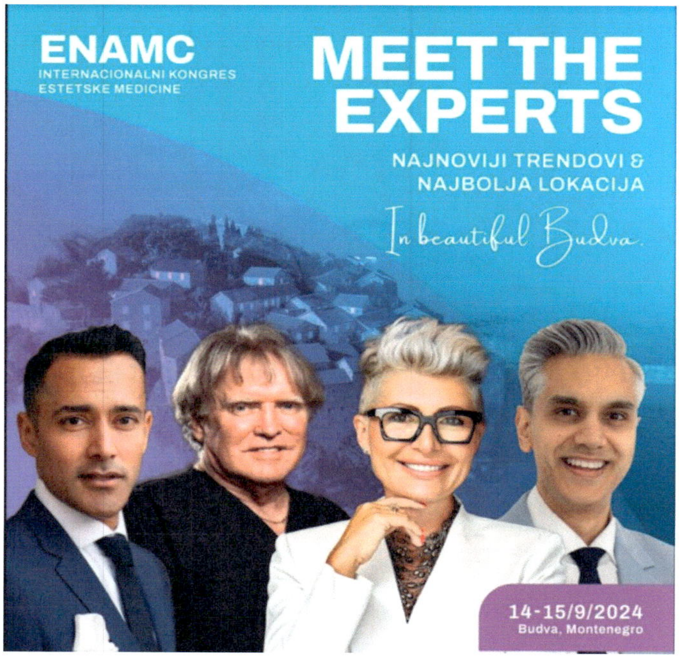

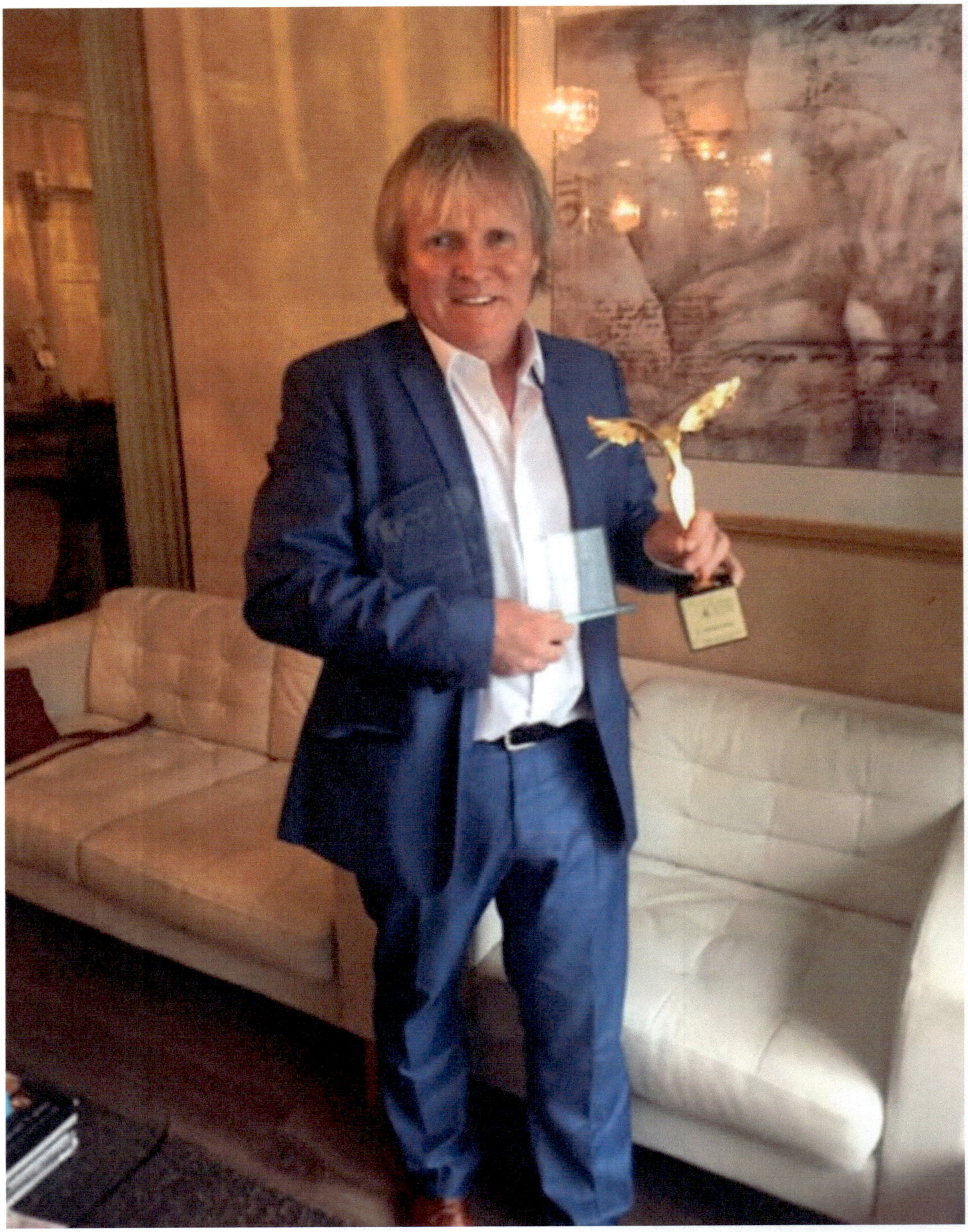

Prof Patrick Treacy's AMEC Award (2016) in Monaco for introducing the Dublin Lift and HELPIR techniques to Aesthetic Medicine

Q17 – What about Stem cells and Tissue Regeneration?

Stem cells, defined by their exceptional ability to **self-renew** and **differentiate into specialized cell types**, stand at the forefront of **regenerative medicine**, offering transformative potential for **tissue repair and replacement**. These versatile cells have driven major advances not only in **aesthetic medicine**—including **skin rejuvenation** and **hair restoration**—but also in **broader clinical applications** such as **organ repair** and the **treatment of complex diseases**. Their integration into innovative protocols, particularly those utilizing **mesenchymal stem cell (MSC)–derived products** such as **Calecim Professional Serum** (in clinical use since 2012), has enabled regenerative strategies that **harness the body's intrinsic healing mechanisms**, producing **natural, long-lasting outcomes** across both **aesthetic** and **therapeutic** domains.

Stem cells are classified according to their **origin** and **differentiation potential**.

- **Embryonic stem cells (ESCs)**, derived from the **inner cell mass of early-stage blastocysts**, are **pluripotent**, capable of differentiating into nearly any cell type in the body. However, their use remains **ethically and legally constrained** due to concerns about **embryo destruction** and **variable international regulations**.
- **Adult (somatic) stem cells**, located in tissues such as **bone marrow**, **adipose tissue**, and **skin**, are generally **multipotent** or **unipotent**, giving rise to specific cell lineages within their native tissue. For example, **hematopoietic stem cells** generate various **blood cell types**. These cells are well established in clinical practice—most notably in **bone marrow transplantation**—owing to their **favorable ethical profile** and **clinical safety record**.
- **Induced pluripotent stem cells (iPSCs)** are **adult somatic cells**, such as **skin fibroblasts**, that have been **genetically reprogrammed** to a **pluripotent state**. They combine the **versatility of ESCs** with **fewer ethical concerns** and **reduced risk of immune rejection** when patient-derived, making them an increasingly powerful platform for **personalized and regenerative therapies**.

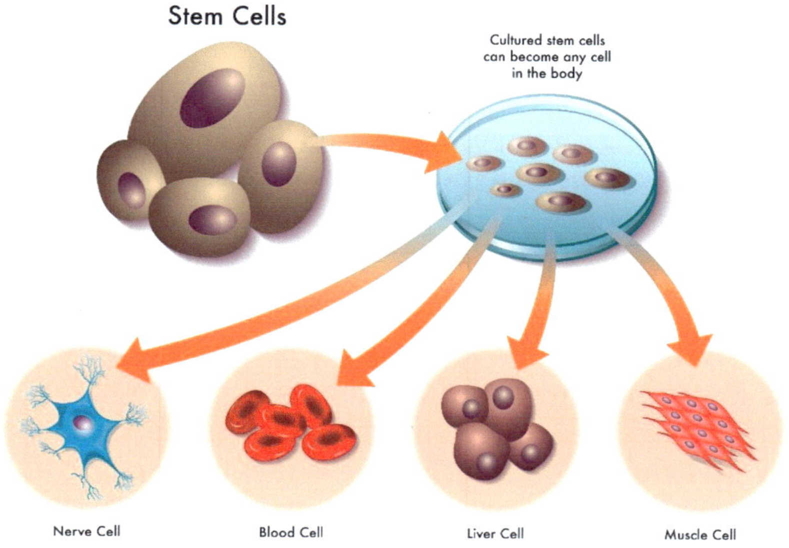

Stem cells are classified according to their **origin** and **differentiation potential. Embryonic stem cells (ESCs)**, derived from the **inner cell mass of early-stage blastocysts**, are **pluripotent**, capable of differentiating into nearly any cell type in the human body. However, their clinical use remains **restricted by ethical considerations** surrounding embryo destruction and **inconsistent regulatory frameworks** across jurisdictions. **Adult (somatic) stem cells**, found in tissues such as **bone marrow**, **adipose tissue**, and **skin**, are generally **multipotent** or **unipotent**, giving rise to specific cell types within their tissue of origin—for instance, **hematopoietic stem cells** that generate blood cells. These cells are widely utilized in established clinical procedures, such as **bone marrow transplantation**, owing to their **lower ethical complexity** and **proven safety profile. Induced pluripotent stem cells (iPSCs)**, produced by **reprogramming adult cells** like skin fibroblasts into a pluripotent state, combine the **developmental versatility of ESCs** with **fewer ethical concerns** and a **reduced risk of immune rejection** when patient-derived, making them a promising foundation for **personalized regenerative therapies**.

The **regenerative capacity of stem cells** operates through **multiple mechanisms**. They can **directly replace** lost or damaged cells by differentiating into specialized types—such as **cardiomyocytes** for cardiac repair or **neurons** for neurological recovery. Equally crucial are their **paracrine effects**, whereby stem cells secrete **growth factors**, **cytokines**, and **extracellular vesicles**, including **exosomes**, which collectively **modulate inflammation**, **promote angiogenesis**, and **stimulate the activity of resident cells**. In **aesthetic applications**, **mesenchymal stem cell (MSC)–derived exosomes**—as found in **Calecim Professional Serum**, introduced clinically in 2012—enhance **collagen synthesis** and **accelerate tissue repair**, improving **skin texture** and **hair follicle function**. In **tissue engineering**, stem cells are seeded onto **biomaterial scaffolds** to guide organized tissue formation, presenting opportunities not only for **aesthetic rejuvenation** but also for **complex organ reconstruction**.

The **clinical applications** of stem cells are **broad and rapidly expanding. Hematopoietic stem cell transplantation** remains a cornerstone therapy for **hematologic malignancies** such as **leukemia** and **lymphoma**, restoring bone marrow function. In **orthopaedics, MSCs** derived from **bone marrow** or **adipose tissue** are used to **regenerate cartilage and bone**, addressing conditions like **osteoarthritis. Cardiac regeneration research** explores stem cell–based repair of **myocardial tissue** following infarction, though **cell retention and integration** remain challenges. In **neurological disorders**, including **Parkinson's disease** and **spinal cord injuries**, stem cells aim to **replace or support** damaged neurons. In **dermatology and wound care**, stem cell–based grafts **accelerate healing** in **chronic wounds** and **burns**, while in **organ bioengineering**, stem cells seeded onto **synthetic or decellularized scaffolds** offer a path toward **lab-grown tissues and organs**, potentially addressing **donor shortages** and **transplant rejection**.

Despite these advances, **stem cell therapies** face **significant challenges**. Ethical constraints surrounding **ESC use**, combined with **regulatory inconsistencies**, continue to limit global application. **Allogeneic stem cell transplants** carry risks of **immune rejection**, while **autologous cells** and **iPSCs** mitigate these concerns but introduce other complexities, such as **production costs** and **technical variability**. The **tumorigenic potential** of pluripotent stem cells, including **teratoma formation**, underscores the need for **rigorous quality control**, **precise differentiation**

protocols, and **stringent safety oversight**. Furthermore, ensuring **standardized, high-quality cell lines** is critical for reproducibility, and the **high cost** of advanced stem cell therapies remains a barrier to widespread accessibility—though emerging **automated culturing** and **bioprocessing innovations** are gradually reducing expenses. The increasing use of **MSC-derived exosomes**, as demonstrated in early **aesthetic protocols**, represents a **cell-free alternative** that minimizes risks such as **immune incompatibility** or **tumorigenesis**, while maintaining potent **regenerative efficacy**.

The **integration of stem cell–based innovations** into **aesthetic protocols**—notably the incorporation of **Calecim Professional Serum** within the **Dublin Lift framework**—has demonstrated how MSC-derived products can **enhance skin and hair rejuvenation**. Rich in **growth factors**, **cytokines**, and **exosomes**, these formulations stimulate **collagen remodeling** and **tissue regeneration**, bridging the fields of **aesthetic enhancement** and **medical repair**. By **2025**, **exosome-based therapies**, inspired by early clinical pioneers, are under investigation for **cartilage repair**, **neurological disorders**, and **chronic wound healing**, reflecting the far-reaching influence of **stem cell applications** in aesthetics. As **regenerative medicine** continues to evolve, stem cells remain central to a **biologically driven paradigm** that redefines both **beauty** and **healing**, shaping a future in which **tissue regeneration** becomes a cornerstone of modern clinical practice.

Applying the Embryonic Stem Cells

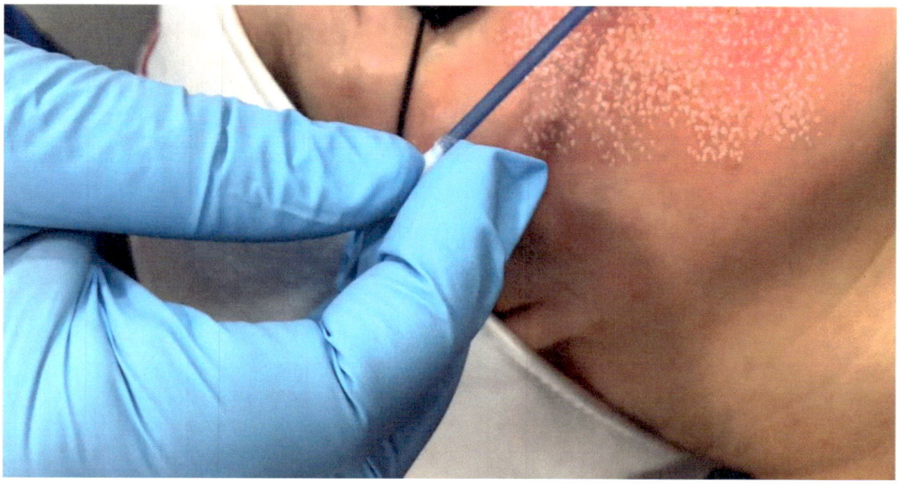

Q18 – What if PRP and Stem cells were used together?

The **PLUS Technique** represents an advanced evolution in regenerative aesthetics, leveraging the biological power of **Platelet-Rich Plasma (PRP)** and key growth factors such as **Transforming Growth Factor Beta (TGF-β)** and **Vascular Endothelial Growth Factor (VEGF)**. These molecules synergistically stimulate collagen synthesis, promote angiogenesis, and enhance cellular turnover, effectively initiating the tissue regeneration process. By accelerating wound healing, PRP shortens recovery time and supports the development of healthier, more resilient tissue, making it particularly effective for repairing skin injuries and post-procedure complications, including those resulting from vascular occlusions. Its autologous nature ensures complete biocompatibility, minimising the risk of adverse reactions while working harmoniously with the body's innate healing mechanisms.

Mesenchymal Stem Cells (MSCs), derived from sources such as umbilical cord or adipose tissue, form a critical component of the PLUS Technique's regenerative framework. These multipotent cells possess the ability to differentiate into various lineages, including fibroblasts and keratinocytes, thereby directly contributing to tissue reconstruction. In addition to their differentiation potential, MSCs secrete a diverse range of bioactive molecules—such as cytokines, growth factors, and exosomes—that modulate inflammation, stimulate angiogenesis, and enhance the function of local cells. This **immunomodulatory capability** plays a key role in balancing inflammatory pathways, preventing excessive immune responses that could otherwise impair healing or increase scarring.

By incorporating **MSC-derived exosome-rich formulations**, a practice established in regenerative aesthetics since 2012, the PLUS Technique significantly amplifies tissue repair and rejuvenation. This integration not only enhances cellular communication and healing efficiency but also delivers consistent, long-term results even in complex cases such as burns or ischemic tissue injury caused by vascular occlusions. Ultimately, the PLUS Technique exemplifies the convergence of cell biology and clinical innovation—offering a scientifically grounded, biologically intelligent approach to achieving accelerated, sustained, and natural tissue regeneration.

2018 What if Stem Cells and PRP were used together

- Platelet-rich plasma (PRP), is a source of various growth factors and signal messengers
- Will act on fibroblasts and stem cells
- Fibroblasts can be stimulated by microneedling or laser resurfacing
- Don't want to do this with occluded damaged tissue
- Add in Stem Cells - mesenchymal or embryonic?

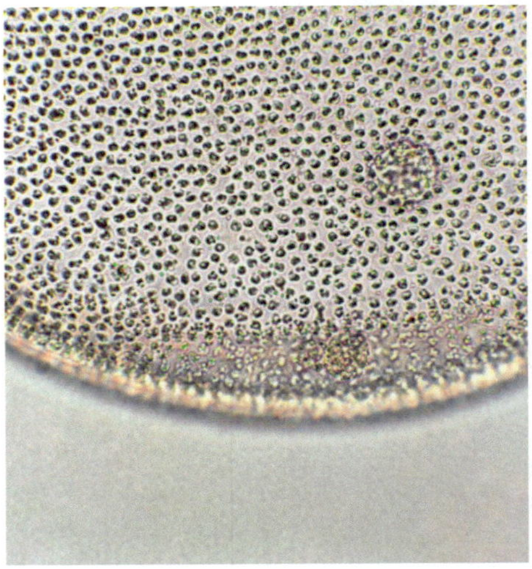

Red-light therapy, typically delivered at a near-red wavelength of **633 nm**, complements **PRP** and **MSCs** by stimulating cellular activity at the mitochondrial level. This wavelength penetrates the dermis to enhance **adenosine triphosphate (ATP)** production, thereby improving cellular energy metabolism, proliferation, and repair functions. By upregulating **collagen gene expression** and accelerating the **wound-healing cascade**, red-light therapy reduces recovery time and optimises tissue repair outcomes. When combined with the growth factors released from PRP and the bioactive signalling molecules secreted by MSCs, it creates a **synergistic regenerative effect**—amplifying collagen remodelling, enhancing angiogenesis, and improving overall tissue viability. This triad of regenerative components underpins the PLUS Technique's effectiveness in treating complex skin injuries, producing superior aesthetic outcomes while minimising downtime.

The integration of **PRP**, **MSCs**, and **red-light therapy** builds upon the foundational principles of the **Dublin Lift**, refining them into a more advanced and targeted system of regenerative aesthetics. By simultaneously addressing multiple dimensions of tissue repair—**collagen synthesis, angiogenesis, inflammation modulation, and cellular stimulation**—the PLUS Technique achieves natural, durable improvements in skin texture, tone, and resilience. Its proven efficacy in managing burns, post-procedural trauma, and **vascular occlusion–related injuries** underscores its versatility, while its **minimally invasive** nature ensures patient comfort and rapid recovery.

As of **June 2025**, the PLUS Technique stands as a testament to the evolution of regenerative medicine—demonstrating how the **strategic combination of biological and phototherapeutic modalities** can transform both aesthetic and reconstructive care. Continuing Dr. **Patrick Treacy's** pioneering legacy, this technique integrates **Platelet-Rich Plasma (PRP)**, **Mesenchymal Stem Cells (MSCs)**, and **red-light therapy** to accelerate healing of skin injuries, burns, and tissue damage, particularly following vascular occlusions. In later developments, **Secretomes** were also incorporated, further enhancing the protocol's regenerative capacity by enriching the cellular communication network essential for optimal tissue restoration.

The **PLUS Technique**, an advanced evolution of the **Dublin Lift**, represents a sophisticated approach to **regenerative aesthetic medicine**. It integrates **Platelet-Rich Plasma (PRP)**, **Mesenchymal Stem Cells (MSCs)**, and **red-light therapy** to accelerate healing in skin injuries, burns, and tissues compromised by **vascular occlusions**. Building on the regenerative foundations of the Dublin Lift, this protocol unites **growth factors**, **bioactive molecules**, and **phototherapeutic stimulation** to promote **epidermal repair**, **collagen induction**, and **enhanced tissue viability**. By offering a **minimally invasive** solution that delivers **natural, long-lasting results** with **rapid recovery**, the PLUS Technique sets a new benchmark for regenerative therapies as of **June 2025**, addressing some of the most complex challenges in dermatological and aesthetic medicine.

Platelet-Rich Plasma (PRP), obtained by centrifuging a patient's blood to isolate and concentrate platelets, serves as a cornerstone of the PLUS Technique. PRP delivers a potent blend of **growth factors**—including **Platelet-Derived Growth Factor (PDGF)**, **Transforming Growth Factor Beta (TGF-β)**, and **Vascular Endothelial Growth Factor (VEGF)**—that stimulate **collagen**

synthesis, **angiogenesis**, and **cellular turnover**, effectively jumpstarting the regenerative process. Its **autologous** nature ensures complete **biocompatibility**, minimising the risk of adverse reactions while supporting the formation of **healthier, more resilient skin**. Within the PLUS framework, PRP functions as a **biological catalyst**, expediting the repair of **burns**, **post-procedural trauma**, and **vascular occlusion–related tissue damage**, where rapid restoration of structural and functional integrity is essential.

Mesenchymal Stem Cells (MSCs), sourced from **umbilical cord**, **adipose tissue**, or **bone marrow**, amplify the regenerative potential of the PLUS Technique through both **differentiation** and **paracrine signalling**. These multipotent cells can transform into fibroblasts and keratinocytes, directly contributing to **dermal and epidermal reconstruction**. More importantly, MSCs secrete **cytokines**, **growth factors**, and **exosomes** that modulate inflammation, stimulate angiogenesis, and enhance the activity of local resident cells. By rebalancing inflammatory cascades, MSCs reduce the likelihood of **fibrosis** and **scarring**, thereby accelerating tissue recovery and improving aesthetic outcomes. The incorporation of **exosome-rich MSC formulations**, first used in aesthetic protocols in **2012**, provides a **cell-free regenerative alternative**—enhancing both safety and efficacy while minimising immunogenic and oncogenic risks.

Red-light therapy, typically delivered at a **near-red wavelength of approximately 633 nm**, complements PRP and MSCs by targeting **mitochondrial activity** within dermal cells. This wavelength penetrates deeply into the skin to **increase adenosine triphosphate (ATP) production)**, thereby enhancing cellular metabolism, proliferation, and overall function. It also **upregulates collagen gene expression**, accelerates **wound healing**, and improves **microcirculatory dynamics**, supporting optimal nutrient and oxygen delivery to regenerating tissues. When combined with the **growth factors** from PRP and the **bioactive signals** from MSCs, red-light therapy produces a **synergistic regenerative environment**, amplifying **collagen remodelling**, reducing **inflammation**, and optimising overall **tissue repair outcomes**.

Together, these three modalities—**PRP**, **MSCs**, and **red-light therapy**—form the foundation of the **PLUS Technique**, marking a pivotal advancement in the evolution of the Dublin Lift. By addressing multiple biological pathways involved in healing and rejuvenation—**collagen induction, angiogenesis, inflammation control, and cellular activation**—the PLUS Technique delivers **natural, durable improvements** in skin quality and resilience. Its adaptability across clinical contexts, including **burns**, **post-procedural damage**, and **ischemic injury**, highlights its **therapeutic versatility**. As regenerative medicine continues to progress, the PLUS Technique exemplifies how **integrative, biologically driven treatments** can redefine aesthetic and reconstructive care, bridging the gap between **medical science and artistry** in modern dermatology.

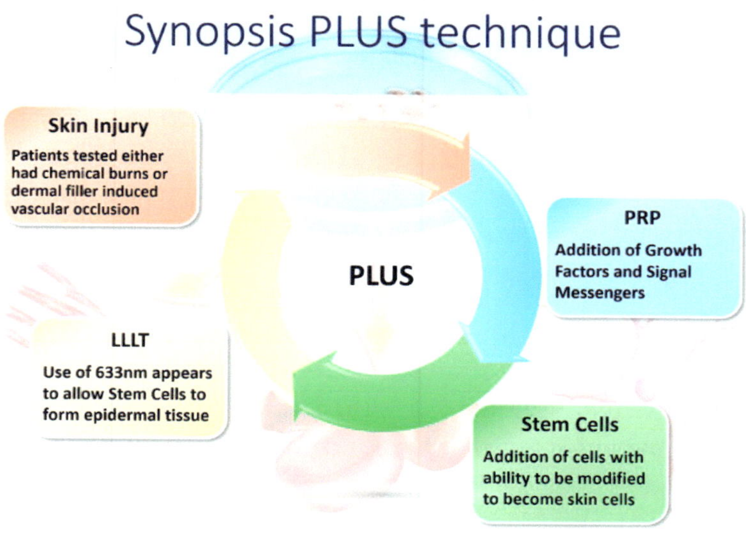

Secretomes refer to the complex ensemble of molecules secreted by cells into the extracellular environment, playing a critical role in **intercellular communication**, **tissue homeostasis**, and **regeneration**. These bioactive components, released by various cell types—including **mesenchymal stem cells (MSCs)**, **immune cells**, and **cancer cells**—encompass a diverse range of molecular species. The secretome is a **heterogeneous mixture** that includes:

- **Proteins and peptides**: Growth factors such as **Vascular Endothelial Growth Factor (VEGF)** and **Transforming Growth Factor Beta (TGF-β)**; cytokines like **Interleukin-6 (IL-6)** and **Tumour Necrosis Factor-alpha (TNF-α)**; and chemokines that regulate **cell proliferation**, **migration**, and **differentiation**.

- **Exosomes (30–150 nm)**: Small extracellular vesicles formed via the endosomal pathway, carrying **mRNAs**, **microRNAs (miRNAs)**, and **proteins** that facilitate intercellular signalling.

- **Microvesicles (100–1000 nm)**: Larger vesicles shed from the plasma membrane, containing **bioactive lipids**, **proteins**, and other signalling molecules.

- **Lipid mediators**: Such as **prostaglandins** and **leukotrienes**, which modulate **inflammatory responses** and **tissue repair**.

- **Metabolites and other factors**: Including **amino acids**, **nucleotides**, and **metabolic byproducts** that influence the local microenvironment and cellular behaviour.

The precise composition of the secretome varies according to the **cell type**, **physiological state** (e.g., hypoxia, inflammation), and **culture conditions**.

The **PLUS Technique** demonstrates exceptional efficacy in treating **chemical and thermal burns**, where rapid **re-epithelialisation** and **collagen repair** are essential for functional recovery. The combined effects of **PRP-derived growth factors**, **MSC secretomes**, and **red-light therapy** minimise scarring, enhance elasticity, and improve overall skin texture over time. In the case of **vascular occlusions**, a known complication of dermal filler procedures, the technique promotes **angiogenesis** through the actions of **VEGF** and **Fibroblast Growth Factor (FGF)**, restoring **oxygenation** and **nutrient delivery** to prevent **tissue necrosis**. Simultaneously, **fibroblast stimulation** aids in **wound closure** and **dermal architecture restoration**. Beyond aesthetics, the PLUS Technique has shown promise in **advanced wound care**, effectively treating **chronic ulcers**, **deep abrasions**, and **post-surgical wounds** with minimal scarring, thereby improving **tissue integrity** across diverse clinical contexts.

The efficacy of the PLUS Technique lies in its **synergistic cellular crosstalk**. PRP-derived **growth factors** and **MSC-derived exosomes** stimulate **fibroblasts** and **keratinocytes** to produce robust **collagen** and **elastin matrices**, reinforcing skin structure and resilience. **Red-light therapy** augments this process by enhancing **mitochondrial ATP production**, which fuels cellular metabolism and accelerates repair. **Inflammation control** is a critical component—while moderate inflammation is essential for healing, excessive responses can exacerbate tissue injury. MSC-secreted **anti-inflammatory cytokines** and PRP's **immune-modulating properties** create a balanced microenvironment that supports efficient tissue regeneration. The **sustained release** of growth factors and **continuous MSC paracrine signalling** ensure **prolonged regenerative activity**, further enhanced by **serial red-light therapy sessions** delivered over several days or weeks.

The **treatment protocol** is meticulously designed for both safety and efficacy. PRP is prepared through **centrifugation** to isolate a concentrated platelet fraction rich in growth factors, while MSCs are processed into **cell concentrates** or **exosome-enriched formulations**. **Red-light therapy**, administered via **LED devices** at approximately **633 nm**, is applied at optimised intervals to stimulate mitochondrial and fibroblast activity. For **burn treatment**, the affected area is thoroughly cleansed before a **PRP–MSC mixture** is applied topically or injected around wound margins, followed by **targeted red-light exposure** to enhance absorption and healing. This integrative approach ensures **comprehensive tissue restoration**, addressing both the biological and structural aspects of repair.

As of **June 2025**, the **PLUS Technique** exemplifies the forefront of **regenerative medicine**, offering a scientifically grounded model of **synergistic, biologically driven healing**. Its expanding applications—spanning from aesthetic rejuvenation to complex wound management—underscore its versatility and transformative potential. By harnessing the body's **innate regenerative capacity**, the PLUS Technique not only advances aesthetic medicine but also lays the foundation for the **next generation of regenerative therapies**, merging precision science with clinical artistry.

Case Report 1: Treating Glycolic Acid Burns with the PLUS Technique

This **case report** presents a detailed account of the **therapeutic management** of a **49-year-old patient** who developed a **severe adverse reaction** following a series of **eighteen glycolic acid facial treatments**. During the final session, the patient experienced acute skin injury that was initially **misdiagnosed as an allergic reaction**. Despite conventional management, the lesion persisted for **three weeks** without visible signs of healing, prompting significant concern regarding the risk of **permanent scarring**.

Methods and Materials:

The patient was subsequently treated using the **PLUS Technique** protocol, which initially employed **Adipose-Derived Stem Cells (ASCs)** and was later refined to incorporate **Umbilical-Derived Stem Cells (USCs)** supplied by **CellResearchCorp, Singapore** [95]. This protocol was designed to **mimic the natural phases of wound healing** through the synergistic application of **Platelet-Rich Plasma (PRP)** and **red-light therapy**, facilitating cellular regeneration and tissue repair. Treatment parameters were **dynamically adjusted** throughout the course of therapy in response to **clinical progress and observed outcomes** [96]. The following section outlines the **specific methodologies and materials** utilized in the treatment process:

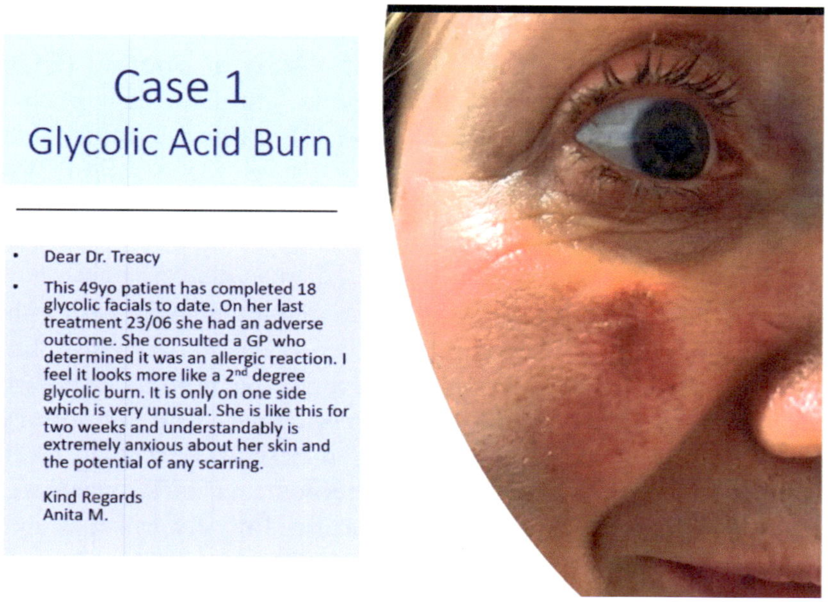

Methods:

- **LED devices for phototherapy** were supplied by *Omnilux* (Birmingham, UK) and *Dermalux TriWave MD*. These systems delivered **red light at a wavelength of 633 nm**, optimized to stimulate **mitochondrial activity, cellular repair, and collagen synthesis**.
- **Umbilical-derived stem cells (USCs)** were **ethically sourced** and **supplied by CellResearchCorp** (Singapore) under **proprietary, Good Manufacturing Practice (GMP)–compliant cultivation protocols**, ensuring cell viability, purity, and safety for clinical application.
- **Platelet-Rich Plasma (PRP)** was **autologously prepared** from the patient's peripheral blood via **centrifugation**, effectively **concentrating platelets and associated growth factors** to enhance tissue regeneration and wound healing.
- **Laser resurfacing** was performed using the **ActiveFX system (Lumenis, Israel)**, calibrated to promote **controlled epithelial regeneration and dermal remodeling**

through fractional ablation, supporting uniform re-epithelialization and improved skin texture.

Stem Cells: Stem cells are undifferentiated, pluripotent cells with the dual capacity for **self-renewal** and differentiation into specialized cell types, including skin, bone, and blood cells. These cells inherently possess the ability to maintain their population while giving rise to multiple cellular lineages. Major sources of stem cells include **embryonic stem cells (ESCs), adult stem cells, perinatal stem cells** (such as those derived from umbilical cord tissue), and **induced pluripotent stem cells (iPSCs)**, each offering distinct therapeutic potentials depending on the clinical application.

Autologous Platelet-Rich Plasma (PRP) Injections: PRP is an **autologous plasma preparation** derived from a patient's own blood via centrifugation, concentrating platelets to deliver a rich profile of growth factors. Upon activation, platelets release key molecules that drive tissue repair, including **Transforming Growth Factor (TGF), Insulin-like Growth Factor (IGF), Platelet-Derived Growth Factor (PDGF), Epidermal Growth Factor (EGF), and Vascular Endothelial Growth Factor (VEGF)**. These factors stimulate **fibroblast-mediated collagen production**, while cytokines such as **Interleukin-1 (IL-1) and Tumor Necrosis Factor-alpha (TNF-α)** support inflammation modulation and tissue regeneration. PRP has become a foundational tool in dermatologic and aesthetic interventions, particularly for accelerating wound healing and skin rejuvenation.

Theory of Effect: Burns and vascular occlusions disrupt normal wound-healing cascades by impairing **clot formation**, thereby limiting the local release of growth factors and cytokines essential for initiating repair. This disruption prevents the normal inflammatory phase, which involves the recruitment of **neutrophils, macrophages, and lymphocytes**, and impedes **keratinocyte proliferation**, leading to maladaptive dermal scarring. Effective wound healing requires the sequential execution of four phases: **hemostasis, inflammation, mesenchymal cell differentiation/proliferation, and re-epithelialization**. Initially, vascular constriction and fibrin clot formation trigger the release of **TGF-β, PDGF, FGF, and EGF**, which recruit inflammatory cells to the wound site. Platelets provide a concentrated source of these growth factors, and PRP amplifies this effect, restoring a **pro-regenerative microenvironment**. Combined with **633 nm red-light therapy**, PRP can **artificially replicate the natural healing cascade**, promoting epidermal repair where the normal process has been disrupted.

Discussion: The decision to implement the **PLUS Technique** in this patient was based on the need to accelerate **skin regeneration** and prevent dermal scarring. The protocol integrates **PRP, mesenchymal stem cells (MSCs), and red-light therapy**, providing a synergistic approach to tissue repair. Initially, **adipose-derived stem cells (ASCs)** were harvested using the **VASER Solta Medical system**, chosen for its efficiency in obtaining viable MSC populations. Following discontinuation of this system, treatment continuity and efficacy were maintained by transitioning to **umbilical-derived stem cells (USCs)** supplied by **CellResearchCorp (Singapore)**, ensuring consistent regenerative potential.

Results: Application of the PLUS Technique facilitated **epidermal tissue regeneration**, resulting in **full clinical recovery within 48 hours**. This rapid outcome underscores the technique's capacity to accelerate regenerative processes.

Conclusion: The patient healed without scarring, indicating that the combined application of **PRP and MSCs**, followed by **633 nm red-light irradiation**, enhances **keratinocyte proliferation** and restores **epithelial tissue integrity**. These findings support the concept of **enhanced epithelial-mesenchymal interactions**, where MSCs and PRP components likely retain postnatal capacities for self-renewal and multilineage differentiation. The outcome demonstrates improved cellular structure, function, and wound repair, aligning with evidence from prior studies in various tissue contexts.

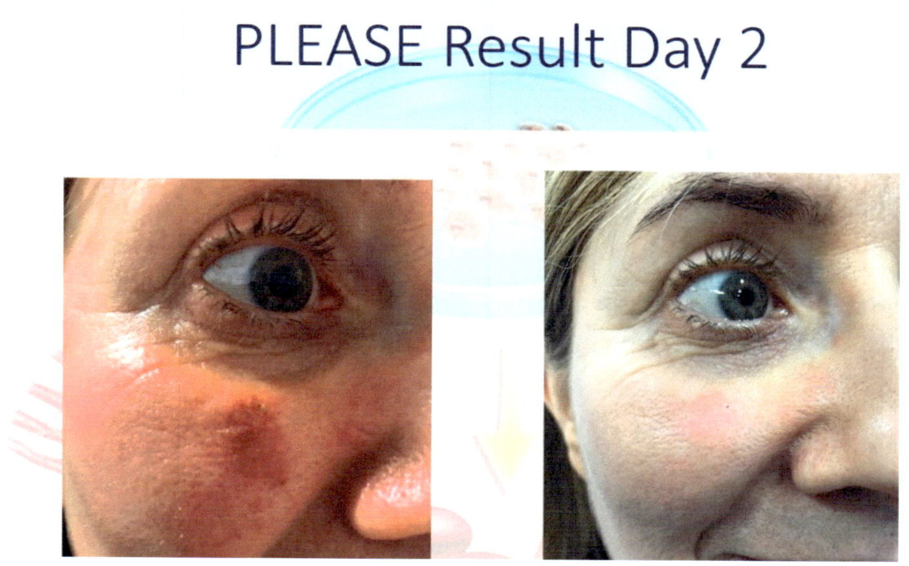

Case Presentation: Treating Grade 3 Full-Thickness Burns Awaiting Skin Graft by PLUS Technique

Patient Presentation:

The patient presented with a **Grade 3 full-thickness burn**, characterized by significant tissue destruction involving the epidermis, dermis, and potential compromise of underlying structures. Such injuries typically require **skin grafting** to facilitate closure and prevent infection. Initial surgical plans were reconsidered following the application of the **PLUS Technique**, which integrates regenerative therapies to accelerate healing and minimize scarring.

Treatment Protocol:

Platelet-Rich Plasma (PRP):

PRP was prepared from the patient's own blood via centrifugation to concentrate platelets, releasing key growth factors, including **Platelet-Derived Growth Factor (PDGF), Transforming Growth Factor Beta (TGF-β), and Vascular Endothelial Growth Factor (VEGF) [76]**. Applied topically or injected around the wound edges, PRP stimulated **fibroblast proliferation**, enhanced **collagen synthesis**, and promoted **angiogenesis**, restoring vascular supply to the damaged tissue [77].

Umbilical Stem Cells (USCs) and Secretomes:

USCs, harvested from **umbilical cord tissue** and expanded in vitro, were combined with their **secretomes**, which contain **exosomes, growth factors (e.g., VEGF, TGF-β), cytokines (e.g., IL-10), and microRNAs [78]**. Secretomes were isolated via ultracentrifugation and delivered paracrine signals that accelerated **epidermal restoration** and modulated inflammation [79]. The anti-inflammatory cytokine **IL-10** and exosomal **miR-21** likely contributed to **scar reduction** and enhanced tissue remodeling [80].

Red-Light Therapy:

Red-light therapy at **633 nm**, delivered using devices such as **Omnilux**, enhanced **cellular metabolism** by stimulating mitochondrial activity and increasing **ATP production [81]**. Applied at **6–8 J/cm² for 10–15 minutes daily**, it synergized with PRP and secretomes to upregulate collagen gene expression (**COL1A1**) and accelerate **wound closure [82]**.

The treatment protocol involved **cleansing the burn site with sterile saline**, applying the **PRP-USC/secretome mixture**, and following with **daily red-light therapy sessions** over 10 days. Adjustments were made based on daily **clinical assessments**, including monitoring for infection and tissue viability.

Outcomes:

Complete recovery was achieved within **10 days**, avoiding the need for grafting. Key contributors to the rapid healing included:

- **Enhanced Collagen Synthesis:** PRP growth factors and secretome-derived TGF-β stimulated fibroblasts to produce a robust **collagen matrix**, restoring dermal integrity [83].
- **Epidermal Restoration:** USC secretomes, particularly exosomes, promoted **re-epithelialization** via delivery of miRNAs that enhanced **keratinocyte proliferation and migration [84]**.
- **Reduced Inflammation and Scarring:** Anti-inflammatory cytokines (e.g., IL-10) and the **photobiomodulatory effects** of red-light therapy minimized excessive inflammatory responses, preventing **hypertrophic scarring**.

Clinical Significance:

This case highlights the **PLUS Technique's efficacy** in managing severe burns, providing a **non-surgical alternative** that reduces typical recovery time (3–6 weeks with grafting) and mitigates associated risks such as **graft rejection and donor-site morbidity [87]**. Integration of secretomes further enhances regenerative potential, making it particularly valuable for younger patients where **preserving aesthetics and function** is critical.

Discussion:

The decision to implement the PLUS Technique was based on its capacity to **accelerate skin healing** and prevent **dermal scarring**. The procedure combines **PRP, MSCs, and red-light therapy**, creating a synergistic regenerative environment. The initial approach utilized **adipose-derived stem cells (ASCs)** harvested using the **VASER Solta Medical system**, selected for its ability to provide high-quality MSC populations in a sterile, bedside setting. Following discontinuation of this system, **umbilical-derived stem cells (USCs)** supplied by **CellResearchCorp, Singapore**, were adopted to maintain **therapeutic continuity and efficacy**.

Theory of Effect:

Grade 3 full-thickness burns and vascular occlusions are marked by **impaired clot formation**, which limits the release of cytokines and growth factors necessary for initiating repair. This disruption prevents the **inflammatory phase**, which typically involves **neutrophil, macrophage, and lymphocyte infiltration**, and results in **keratinocyte deficiency**, impairing epidermal regeneration. Consequently, maladaptive dermal scarring often occurs. Effective wound healing relies on **four sequential phases**:

1. **Rapid hemostasis** – vascular constriction and fibrin clot formation, releasing growth factors such as **TGF-β, PDGF, FGF, and EGF**.
2. **Inflammation** – recruitment of immune cells to the wound site.
3. **Mesenchymal cell differentiation/proliferation** – fibroblast activation and matrix remodeling.
4. **Prompt re-epithelialization** – keratinocyte proliferation and restoration of epidermal integrity.

The PLUS Technique **artificially restores this cascade**, utilizing PRP and MSCs to supply concentrated growth factors and secretomes, while red-light therapy enhances **cellular metabolism**, collectively promoting accelerated healing and reducing the risk of scarring.

For successful wound healing, all **four phases**—hemostasis, inflammation, proliferation, and re-epithelialization—must occur in a **precisely defined sequence** and within an appropriate temporal framework, a process often **disrupted in severe burn injuries**. The **PLUS Technique** accelerates re-epithelialization and collagen repair, minimizing scarring and improving skin texture through the **synergistic action** of PRP's growth factors, MSC-derived anti-inflammatory secretomes, and red-light therapy's cellular stimulation.

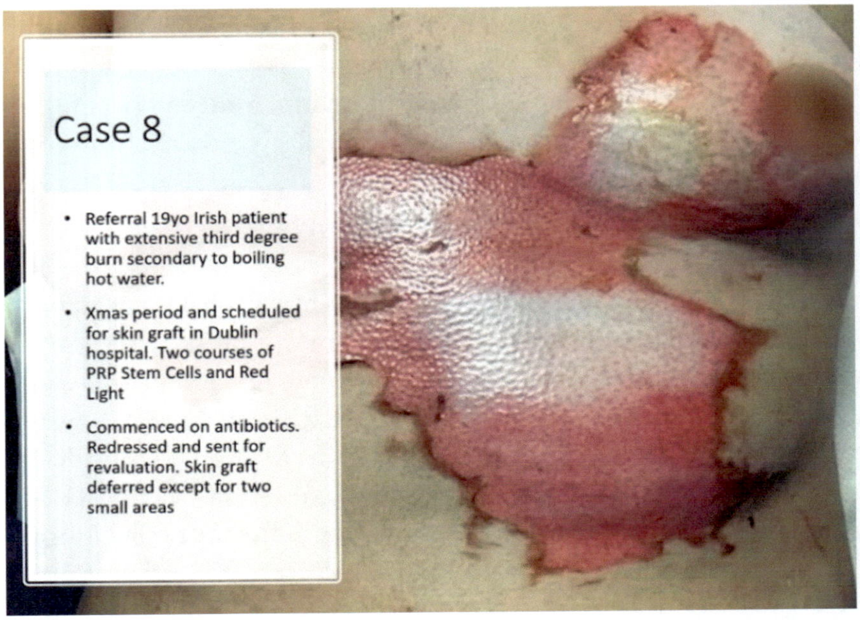

In cases of **vascular occlusion**, a common complication of dermal filler procedures, the PLUS Technique **promotes angiogenesis**, restoring oxygenation and nutrient delivery to prevent necrosis. Simultaneously, fibroblast stimulation supports **wound closure** and the restoration of dermal architecture. The protocol's applications extend to **advanced wound care**, effectively addressing chronic wounds and deep abrasions while minimizing scarring.

The treatment protocol is meticulously designed for **maximized regenerative efficacy**:

- **PRP** is isolated via centrifugation to concentrate platelets and growth factors.
- **MSCs** are processed into cell concentrates or exosome-rich formulations to provide paracrine signaling and anti-inflammatory support.
- **Red-light therapy** is delivered via LED devices at optimized intervals to enhance mitochondrial activity, collagen synthesis, and cellular proliferation.

For **burn injuries**, the damaged area is first cleaned, then a **PRP/MSC mixture** is applied topically or injected around the wound margins, followed by **red-light exposure**. In **vascular occlusion cases**, the PRP/MSC solution may be administered **intradermally** or applied following **microneedling**, with subsequent red-light therapy further enhancing tissue repair and angiogenesis.

Post-treatment care includes additional red-light sessions over the following days, along with protective measures such as **wound dressings** and **sun avoidance**, ensuring optimal healing and minimizing the risk of complications.

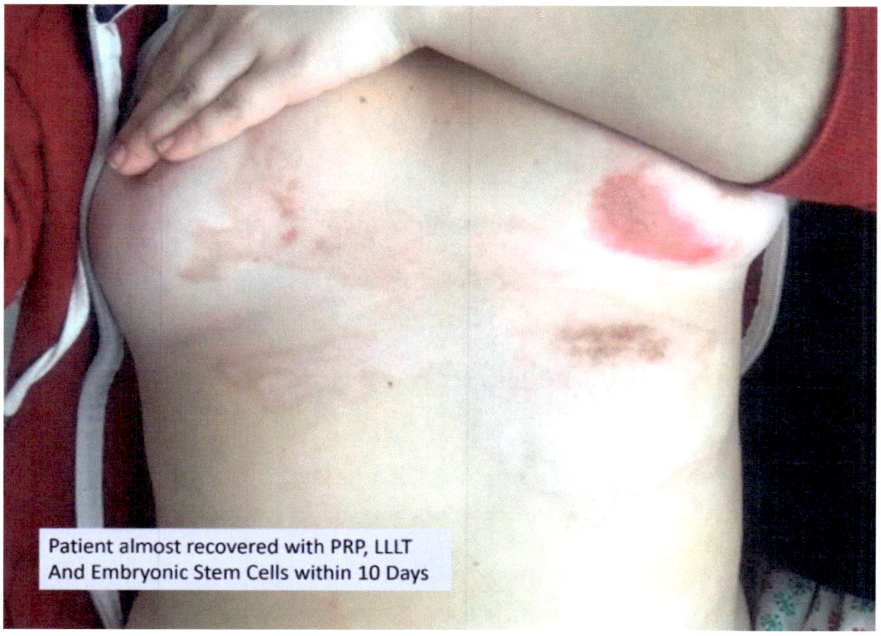

Conclusion

The case of a **21-year-old patient** who sustained a **Grade 3 hot water burn** and achieved complete recovery with the **PLUS Technique** underscores the protocol's potential as an innovative alternative to traditional surgical interventions, such as skin grafting. The following analysis details the components of the PLUS Technique—**Platelet-Rich Plasma (PRP), Umbilical Stem Cells with secretomes, and red-light therapy**—and their roles in facilitating **full recovery within 10 days**.

Case Presentation – Dermal Filler Vascular Occlusion:

A **23-year-old patient** presented with a **vascular occlusion** following dermal filler injection, referred to the author on **day four post-procedure**. She received **two doses of 1500 IU hyaluronidase** over the subsequent days to dissolve the obstructing filler. The **PLUS Technique** was then applied, incorporating PRP, **umbilical MSCs**, and **red-light therapy** using Omnilux and Dermalux TriWave MD devices. Treatment resulted in **complete recovery within 10 days**, with **no scarring**, demonstrating the technique's efficacy in accelerating tissue repair.

Clinical Benefits of the PLUS Technique:

The PLUS Technique offers multiple advantages:

- **Accelerated Healing:** Faster granulation, earlier re-epithelialization, and reduced pain facilitate quicker tissue restoration.
- **Minimized Scarring:** By promoting uniform collagen deposition, the protocol achieves smoother, healthier skin with superior aesthetic outcomes.

- **Reduced Complications:** The combined approach addresses **inflammation, ischemia, and cellular stress**, thereby decreasing the risk of infection, necrosis, and prolonged inflammatory responses.

Mechanisms of Action:

The therapeutic synergy of the PLUS Technique is underpinned by **cellular crosstalk**:

- **PRP growth factors** and **MSC-derived exosomes** stimulate fibroblasts and keratinocytes to produce robust **collagen and elastin matrices**.
- **Red-light therapy** enhances these effects by increasing **ATP production** and cellular activity, amplifying tissue repair and collagen remodeling.
- **Anti-inflammatory cytokines** from MSCs, combined with PRP's immunomodulatory support, prevent excessive inflammation, ensuring efficient and controlled healing.
- The **slow, sustained release** of growth factors and ongoing MSC paracrine signaling prolong regenerative activity, reinforced by **repeated red-light therapy sessions**.

Together, these coordinated mechanisms enable the PLUS Technique to achieve **rapid, scar-free tissue repair**, even in complex cases such as severe burns and vascular occlusions, highlighting its transformative potential in **regenerative aesthetic and reconstructive medicine**.

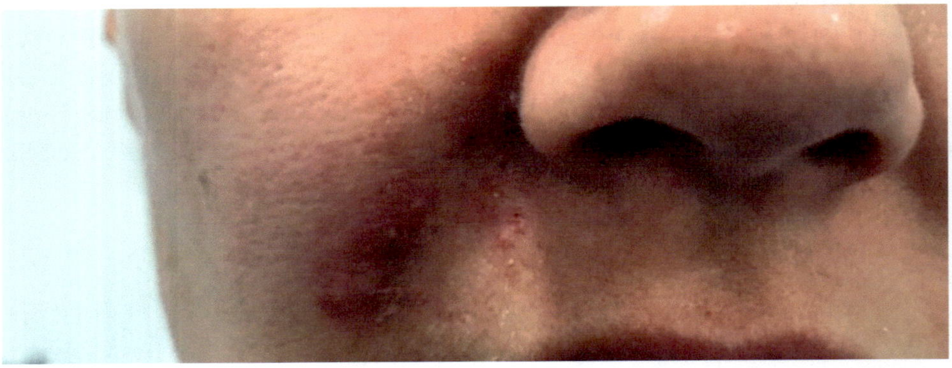

The broader field of **regenerative medicine**, exemplified by the **PLUS Technique** and its use of **mesenchymal stem cells (MSCs)** and **exosome-rich formulations**—notably via **Calecim Professional Serum** since 2012—is poised for transformative advancements. **Induced pluripotent stem cells (iPSCs)** provide patient-specific cell lines for disease modeling and therapeutic applications, minimizing the risk of immune rejection and enabling **personalized regenerative solutions** tailored to individual patients.

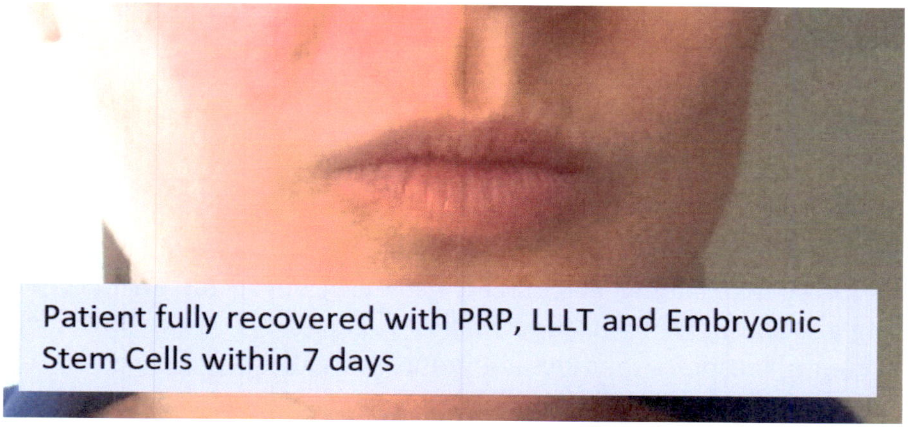

The **PLUS Technique**—integrating **Platelet-Rich Plasma (PRP)**, **Mesenchymal Stem Cells (MSCs)**, and **red-light therapy**—serves as a model for **synergistic, biologically driven healing**, with applications extending beyond aesthetics to **advanced wound care**. By harnessing the body's intrinsic regenerative capacity, it delivers **rapid, natural, and durable outcomes**, establishing a foundation for **next-generation regenerative therapies**. As of June 2025, advances in stem cell biology, biomaterials, and gene editing are expanding regenerative medicine toward innovative solutions for complex medical conditions, from wound repair to organ replacement, transforming both clinical practice and patient care.

Clinical Benefits: The PLUS Technique accelerates healing by reducing pain, promoting faster granulation, and enabling earlier re-epithelialisation, resulting in **smoother, healthier skin**. By minimizing scar formation and promoting **uniform collagen deposition**, it achieves superior aesthetic results, particularly in **complex injury scenarios**. Its multi-faceted approach—combining growth factors, MSC signaling, and photobiomodulation—reduces complications such as infection, necrosis, and prolonged inflammation by simultaneously addressing **cellular stress, ischemia, and inflammatory cascades**. Cellular crosstalk underpins this synergy: **PRP growth factors** and **MSC-derived exosomes** stimulate fibroblasts and keratinocytes to produce robust collagen and elastin matrices, while **red-light therapy** enhances these responses via increased ATP production. Anti-inflammatory cytokines from MSCs, together with PRP's immunomodulatory effects, prevent excessive inflammation, ensuring efficient tissue repair. Sustained growth factor release and ongoing MSC paracrine signaling, reinforced by repeated red-light sessions, maintain a **prolonged regenerative environment**.

Future Directions: The principles of the PLUS Technique align with emerging trends in regenerative medicine. **Induced pluripotent stem cells (iPSCs)** enable the generation of patient-specific cell lines for disease modeling and therapy, mitigating immune rejection risks and supporting **personalized regenerative solutions**. Gene-editing technologies such as **CRISPR/Cas9** offer potential for correcting genetic defects in stem cells prior to transplantation, addressing inherited conditions. Combination therapies integrating stem cells with growth factors, exosomes, or biomaterials are under investigation to **maximize tissue repair synergy**, exemplifying the approach pioneered by the PLUS Technique. Ongoing clinical trials and translational research continue to refine protocols, balancing **safety concerns**—including the tumorigenic potential of pluripotent stem cells—with therapeutic efficacy for conditions ranging from degenerative diseases to traumatic injuries. Although challenges remain, including ethical considerations, immune compatibility, and cost, advances in cell-culturing and **exosome-based therapies** are improving accessibility, reproducibility, and outcomes.

Conclusion: By combining PRP, MSCs, and red-light therapy, the PLUS Technique provides a **robust framework for regenerative aesthetics** and advanced wound care. Its biologically driven approach achieves rapid, natural, and durable outcomes, advancing the field of aesthetic medicine while offering a blueprint for future regenerative therapies. As regenerative medicine continues to evolve, this strategy inspires solutions for complex medical challenges—from wound repair to tissue regeneration—reshaping clinical practice and enhancing patient care.

Q19 – How Does Red Light Work in Epidermal Repair?

Red light therapy (RLT), typically administered at wavelengths near **633 nm** or within the **red/near-infrared spectrum (600–700 nm)**, is a key component of regenerative aesthetic protocols such as the **PLUS Technique**. RLT enhances **epidermal repair**, modulates **growth factor activity**, and optimizes **cellular function**. The light penetrates tissues and is absorbed by **cytochrome c oxidase** in the mitochondria, stimulating **ATP production** and improving overall **cellular metabolism**. This increase in cellular energy promotes the **proliferation, migration, and viability** of critical cell types, including **keratinocytes** and **fibroblasts**, establishing a robust foundation for tissue repair.

Within the PLUS Technique, which builds upon the regenerative framework of the **Dublin Lift**, RLT acts **synergistically** with **Platelet-Rich Plasma (PRP)** and **Mesenchymal Stem Cells (MSCs)** to accelerate healing in **skin injuries, burns, and tissues affected by vascular occlusions**. This integrated approach delivers **rapid, natural, and durable outcomes**, enhancing both functional recovery and aesthetic results.

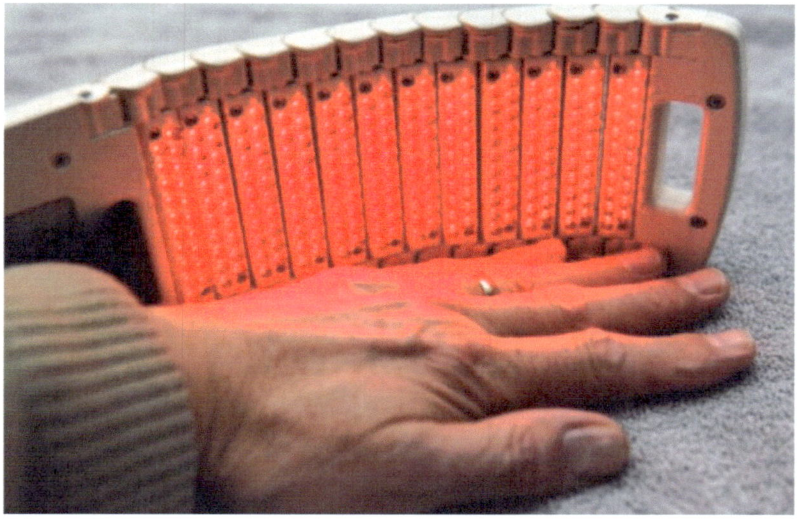

The therapeutic efficacy of **red-light therapy (RLT)** lies in its ability to regulate **growth factors** that are critical for tissue regeneration. By increasing intracellular energy, RLT enhances cellular capacity to **synthesize and release growth factors** such as **Vascular Endothelial Growth Factor (VEGF)**, **Transforming Growth Factor Beta (TGF-β)**, and **Fibroblast Growth Factor (FGF)**. These molecules orchestrate **angiogenesis, collagen remodeling, and re-epithelialisation**, thereby accelerating wound healing and improving skin texture in conditions such as burns or post-vascular occlusion injury. Within the **PLUS Technique**, RLT amplifies the regenerative effects of **PRP-derived growth factors** and **MSC bioactive signals**, creating a **synergistic microenvironment** that promotes robust tissue repair. For example, in the management of chemical burns or chronic wounds, RLT facilitates **uniform collagen deposition**, minimizing scarring and optimizing aesthetic outcomes; in hair restoration, it enhances **follicle vitality**, complementing the actions of MSC-derived exosomes.

RLT also plays a pivotal role in **modulating inflammation and oxidative stress**, establishing an optimal environment for tissue regeneration. It upregulates **antioxidant enzymes** such as **superoxide dismutase (SOD)** and **catalase**, while regulating **NF-κB activity**, thereby balancing inflammatory responses and preventing excessive inflammation that could delay healing or increase scar formation. This **anti-inflammatory effect** is particularly valuable within the PLUS Technique, where it complements MSC secretion of **anti-inflammatory cytokines** and PRP's immune-modulatory support, reducing complications such as infection or prolonged inflammation in complex scenarios like vascular occlusions. The cumulative result is **accelerated granulation, earlier re-epithelialisation, and reduced downtime**, yielding smoother, healthier skin post-injury.

In the PLUS Technique protocol, RLT is delivered via **LED-based devices** at approximately **633 nm**, with optimized exposure times following the application of **PRP/MSC mixtures**, administered either topically or via **intradermal injection**, especially for burns or post-vascular occlusion recovery. **Aftercare** includes additional RLT sessions over subsequent days, combined with protective measures such as wound dressings and sun avoidance, to maximize tissue recovery. By enhancing **cellular crosstalk**—where PRP growth factors and MSC-derived exosomes stimulate fibroblasts and keratinocytes, while RLT increases ATP production—this approach establishes a **sustained regenerative environment**.

As regenerative medicine continues to advance in June 2025, the integration of RLT with PRP and MSCs in protocols like the PLUS Technique represents a **gold standard for synergistic healing**, with applications extending beyond aesthetics to **advanced wound care**. Emerging strategies, including the combination of RLT with **personalized stem cell therapies** or **gene-edited cell lines**, hold the potential to further enhance regenerative outcomes, transforming both aesthetic and medical clinical practice.

Q20 – What is Dr. Patrick Treacy's theory regarding the reversal of epithelial–mesenchymal transition (EMT) in the presence of mesenchymal stem cells (MSCs):

Red-light therapy (RLT), typically administered at wavelengths near **633 nm** or within the **red/near-infrared range (600–700 nm)**, is a critical component of regenerative aesthetic protocols such as the **PLUS Technique**. It enhances **epidermal repair and tissue stability** by modulating cellular phenotypes through its influence on **epithelial–mesenchymal transition (EMT)** and **mesenchymal-to-epithelial transition (MET)**. EMT, wherein epithelial cells lose polarity and adhesion to acquire migratory, mesenchymal traits, is essential for embryogenesis and wound healing but can contribute to **pathological scarring or fibrosis** if dysregulated. Conversely, MET restores epithelial characteristics, promoting **stable tissue architecture**. Within the PLUS Technique—which integrates **Platelet-Rich Plasma (PRP)**, **Mesenchymal Stem Cells (MSCs)**, and RLT to accelerate healing of burns, skin injuries, and post-vascular occlusion damage—RLT synergizes with MSCs to **shift cellular signaling away from excessive EMT toward MET**, fostering robust epithelial repair and minimizing scarring.

RLT's mechanism begins with absorption by **cytochrome c oxidase** in the mitochondria, enhancing **ATP production** and thereby improving the **metabolism, proliferation, and migration** of cells such as keratinocytes and fibroblasts. This increase in cellular energy supports the **synthesis and release of growth factors**, including **Vascular Endothelial Growth Factor (VEGF)**, **Transforming Growth Factor Beta (TGF-β)**, and **Fibroblast Growth Factor (FGF)**, which coordinate **angiogenesis, collagen remodeling, and re-epithelialisation**. Within the PLUS Technique, these growth factors complement **PRP's regenerative signals**, accelerating wound healing. RLT also upregulates **antioxidant enzymes** such as **superoxide dismutase (SOD)** and **catalase**, while modulating **NF-κB activity** to balance inflammatory responses, creating a **favorable microenvironment for tissue regeneration**. By mitigating excessive inflammation, RLT prevents prolonged EMT—which can delay epithelial closure or cause fibrotic changes—thus supporting MET and **stable epithelial integrity**.

MSCs further enhance RLT's effects by secreting a **potent secretome** of cytokines, exosomes, and growth factors that guide cellular behavior. In the presence of RLT, MSCs produce "**epithelial-friendly**" growth factors such as **Epidermal Growth Factor (EGF)**, promoting **keratinocyte proliferation and tight junction formation**, thereby reinforcing MET. MSCs also modulate **TGF-β pathways**, a key regulator of EMT, shifting signaling toward isoforms that **stabilize epithelial phenotypes** in the later phases of healing. Through secretion of **anti-inflammatory cytokines** like IL-10 and exosomes, MSCs further reduce chronic inflammation, preventing mesenchymal dominance and fostering an **epithelial-supportive microenvironment**. Concurrently, RLT enhances **extracellular matrix (ECM) organization**, encouraging fibroblasts and keratinocytes to deposit **collagen, fibronectin, and laminin-rich matrices**, which provide the structural scaffold necessary for **epithelial adhesion and barrier function**.

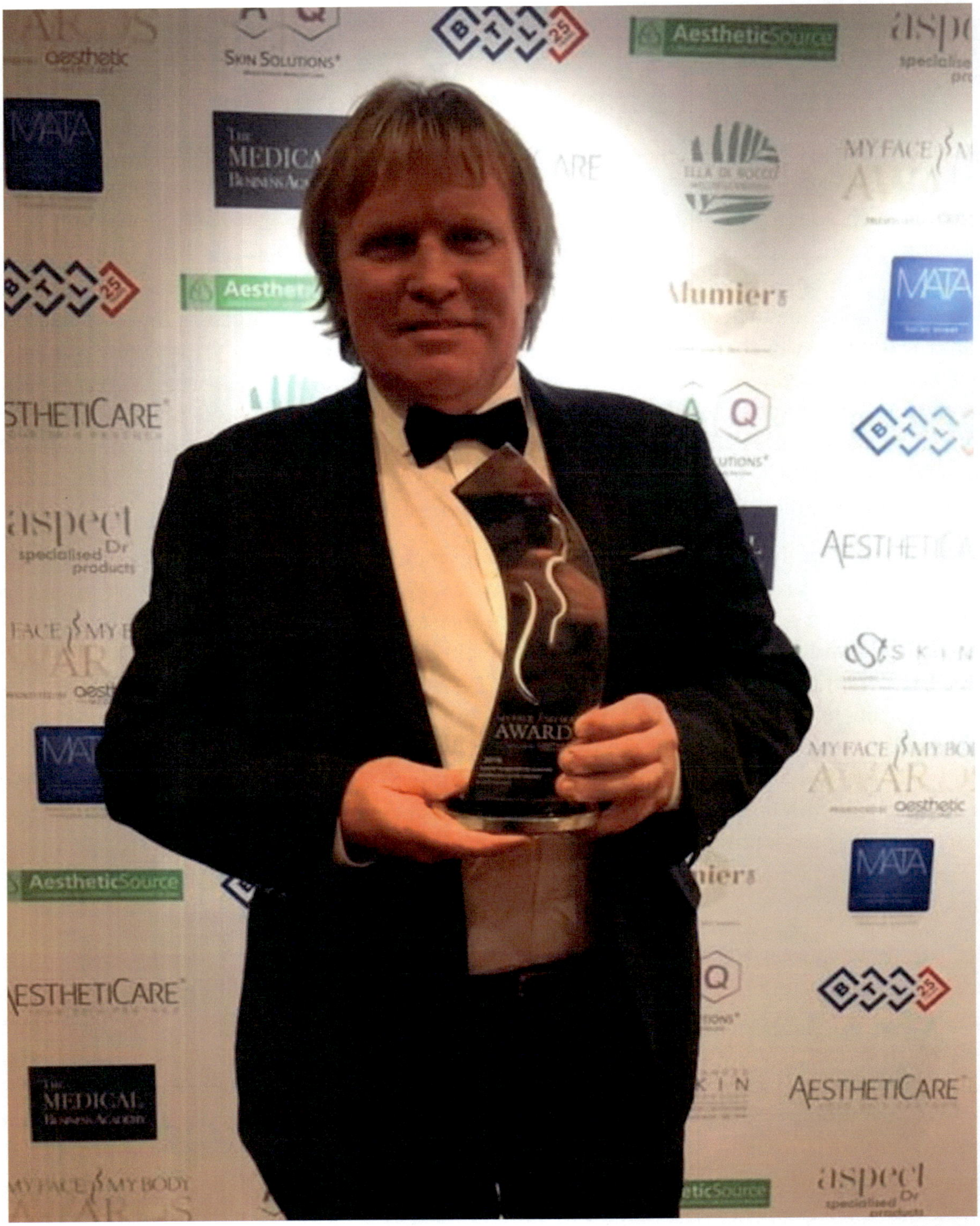

Prof Patrick Treacy receiving the MyFaceMyBody Award (2018) in London for research relating to the HELPIR and PLUS techniques.

The **practical implications** of this synergistic approach are profound for **skin healing and aesthetic rejuvenation**. In burn treatment, the combination of **RLT, MSCs, and PRP** accelerates **re-epithelialisation**, minimizes scarring, and enhances skin texture by promoting **MET**, ensuring faster and more complete epidermal closure. For **post-vascular occlusion damage**, often a complication of dermal fillers, this strategy restores tissue integrity by enhancing **angiogenesis** and **fibroblast activity**, while preventing excessive **EMT-driven fibrosis**. In aesthetic contexts, modulating EMT preserves structural integrity in aging or damaged skin, reinforcing **epithelial adhesion and barrier function**, and reducing complications such as **hypertrophic scarring** or **hyperpigmentation**, thereby maintaining robust tissue homeostasis.

The treatment protocol integrates **RLT** with **PRP** and **MSC applications**, typically involving **topical or intradermal delivery of PRP/MSC mixtures**, followed by **633 nm red-light exposure via LED devices**. Aftercare includes additional RLT sessions and protective measures, such as **wound dressings** and **sun avoidance**, to optimize recovery. By leveraging **RLT's ATP-enhancing effects** and MSC-driven **paracrine signalling**, the technique creates a **high-energy, balanced microenvironment** that promotes **MET over unchecked EMT**, ensuring ordered epithelial regeneration and stable tissue repair.

Mechanisms of Action:

RLT's therapeutic efficacy stems from its ability to penetrate tissues and be absorbed by **cytochrome c oxidase** in mitochondria, boosting **ATP production** and enhancing the **metabolism, proliferation, and migration** of cells such as **keratinocytes** and **fibroblasts**. This increased cellular energy facilitates the synthesis and release of "**epithelial-friendly**" growth factors, including **Epidermal Growth Factor (EGF)**, which promotes keratinocyte proliferation and **tight junction formation**, supporting MET. RLT also modulates **TGF-β pathways**, a key regulator of EMT, favoring isoforms that stabilize epithelial phenotypes in later healing phases and shifting cells away from migratory, mesenchymal states. Additionally, RLT upregulates **antioxidant enzymes** such as **superoxide dismutase (SOD)** and **catalase**, while modulating **NF-κB activity** to balance inflammation, preventing chronic inflammatory states that drive excessive EMT.

MSCs enhance these effects by secreting a **potent secretome** of cytokines, exosomes, and growth factors that guide cellular behavior toward MET. Anti-inflammatory cytokines, such as **IL-10**, reduce chronic inflammation, creating an **epithelial-friendly microenvironment**. MSCs also secrete **collagen, fibronectin, and laminin-rich extracellular matrices (ECM)**, providing the structural scaffold required for epithelial cells to form tight junctions rather than remain migratory. Within the PLUS Technique, the synergy of RLT, MSCs, and **PRP-derived growth factors** (e.g., **PDGF, TGF-β, VEGF**) stimulates fibroblasts and keratinocytes to produce **robust collagen and elastin matrices**, enhancing tissue repair and reinforcing epithelial integrity, thereby reducing the risk of fibrotic responses or abnormal scarring.

Clinical Applications and Outcomes:

In burn cases, this integrated approach accelerates re-epithelialisation, stabilizes the epidermis, and achieves faster, more complete healing with minimal scarring. For **post-vascular occlusion**

damage, it promotes angiogenesis and fibroblast activity, restoring dermal architecture while preventing EMT-driven fibrosis. In **aesthetic rejuvenation**, modulating EMT improves epithelial cell adhesion, tight junction formation, and barrier function, countering structural decline associated with aging or chronic skin damage and resulting in smoother, healthier skin.

By **leveraging RLT's ATP-enhancing and anti-inflammatory properties** alongside MSC paracrine signaling, the PLUS Technique creates a **high-energy, regenerative microenvironment** that favors MET over uncontrolled EMT, ensuring stable tissue repair. Rooted in the **Dublin Lift's regenerative framework**, this approach, as of June 2025, establishes a foundation for future therapies, synergizing with innovations such as **induced pluripotent stem cells (iPSCs)** and **gene editing** to enhance tissue regeneration across **aesthetic and medical applications**.

Q 21 – What is Chemical Signalling?

Chemical signaling in cells is the process by which cells communicate through chemical molecules to transmit information, coordinate activities, and regulate physiological functions. This process involves **signaling molecules**—such as hormones, neurotransmitters, cytokines, and growth factors—released by a source cell, which bind to **specific receptors** on or within a target cell. Binding initiates a cascade of intracellular events known as **signal transduction**, which can alter gene expression, metabolism, or cell behavior, including **proliferation, differentiation, or apoptosis**.

There are several types of chemical signaling:

- **Autocrine:** The cell signals itself.
- **Paracrine:** The cell signals nearby cells.
- **Endocrine:** Signals are sent to distant cells via the bloodstream.
- **Juxtacrine:** Signals occur through direct cell-to-cell contact.

Exosomes, small lipid vesicles measuring 30–150 nm, play a crucial role in paracrine signaling by delivering molecular cargos—such as microRNAs (miRNAs), proteins, and lipids—to target cells. These vesicles modulate cellular responses, for instance by **promoting tissue repair**, regulating inflammation, or enhancing cell survival. By efficiently delivering signaling molecules to specific cells, exosomes can amplify biological effects, such as **anti-inflammatory responses** or activation of survival pathways.

In summary, **chemical signaling is a fundamental mechanism of cellular communication**, driving processes essential for **development, tissue homeostasis, and disease response**. It provides a versatile framework for coordinating complex cellular networks, both under normal physiological conditions and in response to injury or stress.

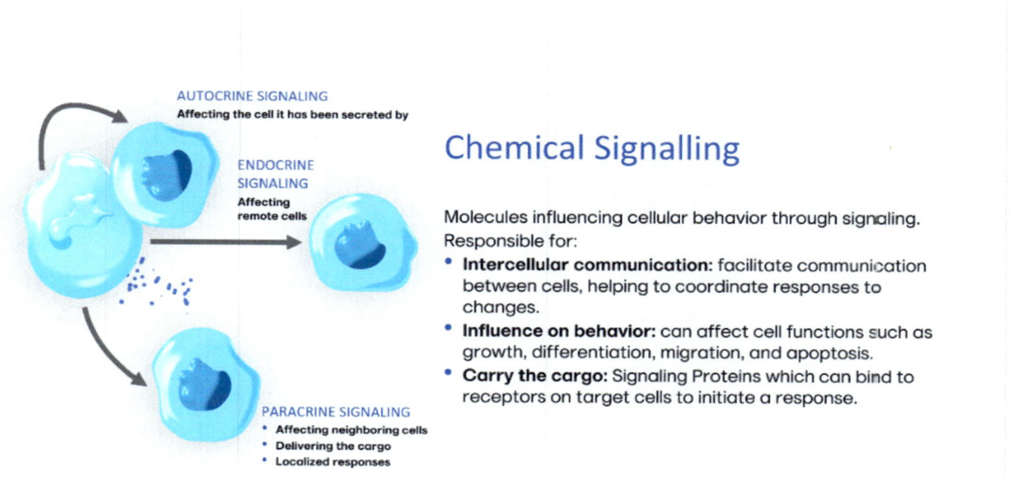

Q 22 – What exactly are Secretomes?

Secretomes, the dynamic collection of molecules secreted by cells, play a central role in intercellular communication and tissue regeneration, making them a cornerstone of regenerative aesthetic protocols such as the PLUS Technique. These secreted factors include **proteins and peptides, extracellular vesicles (e.g., exosomes), lipid mediators, and other bioactive molecules** that orchestrate complex biological processes, including wound healing, immune modulation, and tissue repair.

In particular, MSC-derived secretomes are rich in **growth factors** such as Vascular Endothelial Growth Factor (VEGF) and Transforming Growth Factor Beta (TGF-β), **cytokines** including IL-6 and TNF-α, and **exosomes** carrying mRNAs and microRNAs, all of which enhance cellular proliferation, migration, and differentiation. Within the PLUS Technique—which integrates **Platelet-Rich Plasma (PRP), Mesenchymal Stem Cells (MSCs), and red-light therapy (RLT)** to address burns, skin injuries, and post-vascular occlusion damage—these secretomes amplify epidermal repair, stimulate collagen synthesis, modulate inflammation, and improve tissue resilience.

This **synergistic interplay**, combining the MSC-derived secretome with PRP's concentrated growth factors and RLT's photobiomodulatory stimulation, replicates and accelerates the natural regenerative cascade. Rooted in the framework of the Dublin Lift, this approach promotes **rapid, natural, and durable outcomes**, advancing both aesthetic and clinical healing by reinforcing tissue integrity, reducing scarring, and restoring optimal skin function.

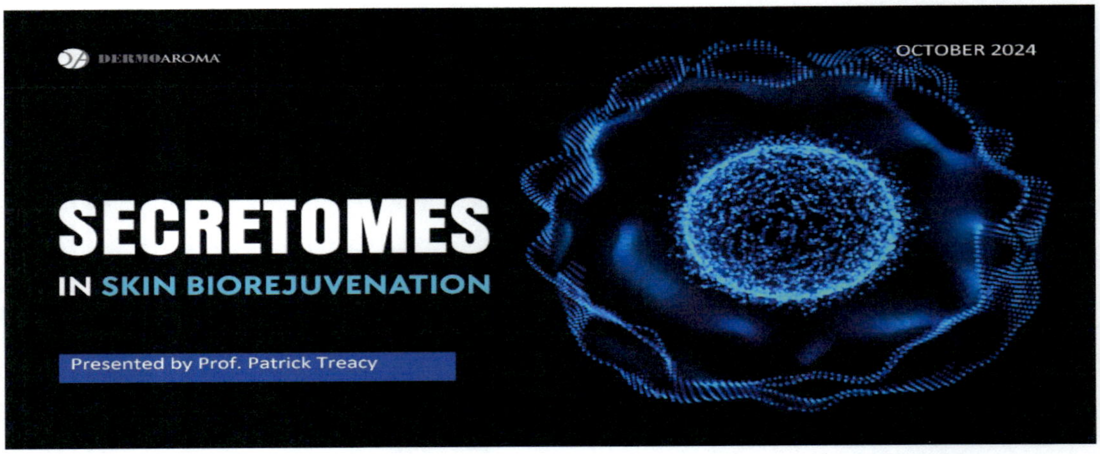

The **composition of secretomes** is highly diverse and tailored to the cell type and its microenvironment. Proteins and peptides, including growth factors and cytokines, regulate inflammation, cell proliferation, and tissue remodelling, driving processes such as **collagen synthesis and angiogenesis**. Extracellular vesicles, particularly **exosomes**, carry proteins, lipids, mRNAs, and microRNAs, facilitating intercellular communication by transferring bioactive signals that modulate cellular behaviour, including promoting **epithelial–mesenchymal transition (EMT)** or its reversal, **mesenchymal-to-epithelial transition (MET)**. Lipid mediators contribute to immune regulation and cell metabolism, while hormones and metabolites further enhance tissue repair. The specific profile of secretomes varies by cell type—**mesenchymal stem cells (MSCs), immune cells, and fibroblasts** each produce distinct secretomes reflecting their physiological roles—and is influenced by environmental conditions such as hypoxia, inflammation, or tissue injury, which dynamically upregulate or downregulate factors to meet healing demands.

In 2021, the author **modified the PLUS Technique** to incorporate **Purosomes** from DermaAroma, derived from bovine colostrum—a rich source of bioactive proteins, growth factors, and immunoglobulins. This addition enhances the technique's regenerative potential, particularly in **skin rejuvenation and hair restoration**, by amplifying the delivery of bioactive molecules that stimulate tissue repair and reduce inflammation. The later PLUS Technique protocol involves applying **PRP/MSC secretome mixtures**, sometimes including Purosomes, either **topically or intradermally**, often following **microneedling**, followed by **red-light therapy (RLT)**. Aftercare includes additional RLT sessions and protective measures, such as wound dressings or scalp care, to optimise outcomes. This combined approach accelerates **re-epithelialisation, collagen synthesis, and angiogenesis** in skin injuries, burns, and post-vascular occlusion damage, while supporting **hair follicle health**. Regulatory oversight for secretome-based therapies, including bovine colostrum-derived products like Purosomes, is evolving to ensure safety and efficacy, with ongoing efforts to standardise isolation and processing methods. As of June 2025, combining secretomes with **biomaterials or gene-editing technologies such as CRISPR/Cas9** promises to further enhance regenerative outcomes, positioning the PLUS Technique as a model for addressing **age-related decline in aesthetic and clinical applications**, from skin rejuvenation to hair restoration.

In the later PLUS Technique, **MSCs remain central** to regenerative efficacy, particularly in **modulating EMT and promoting MET** to stabilise epithelial integrity. MSCs secrete growth factors such as **VEGF and TGF-β**, which, in synergy with PRP's growth factors, stimulate fibroblast and keratinocyte activity, enhancing **collagen and elastin production** for robust **extracellular matrix (ECM) organisation**. Exosomes, enriched with microRNAs, further guide cellular phenotypes, supporting MET and preventing excessive EMT-driven fibrosis or scarring in burns and vascular occlusion recovery. **Anti-inflammatory cytokines** like IL-10 reduce chronic inflammation, creating an epithelial-friendly microenvironment that complements RLT's anti-inflammatory effects, which upregulate antioxidant enzymes and modulate NF-κB activity.

RLT also boosts ATP production, enhancing MSC secretome output, **amplifying growth factor release and cellular metabolism**, and creating a synergistic healing environment that accelerates **re-epithelialisation** and minimises complications such as hypertrophic scarring or hyperpigmentation. The practical implications of secretomes in the PLUS Technique are profound: in **burn treatment**, MSC secretomes combined with PRP and RLT accelerate wound closure and collagen repair, reducing scarring and improving skin texture. In **post-vascular occlusion damage**, secretome-derived angiogenic signals restore tissue perfusion, while anti-inflammatory factors prevent necrosis. In aesthetic applications, secretomes reinforce **skin barrier function and structural integrity**, countering age-related decline.

As regenerative medicine advances in June 2025, the integration of **bovine colostrum-derived secretomes**, with their rich repertoire of bioactive molecules, sets a foundation for future therapies, expanding the PLUS Technique's potential across **skin and hair restoration, advanced wound care, and aesthetic medicine**.

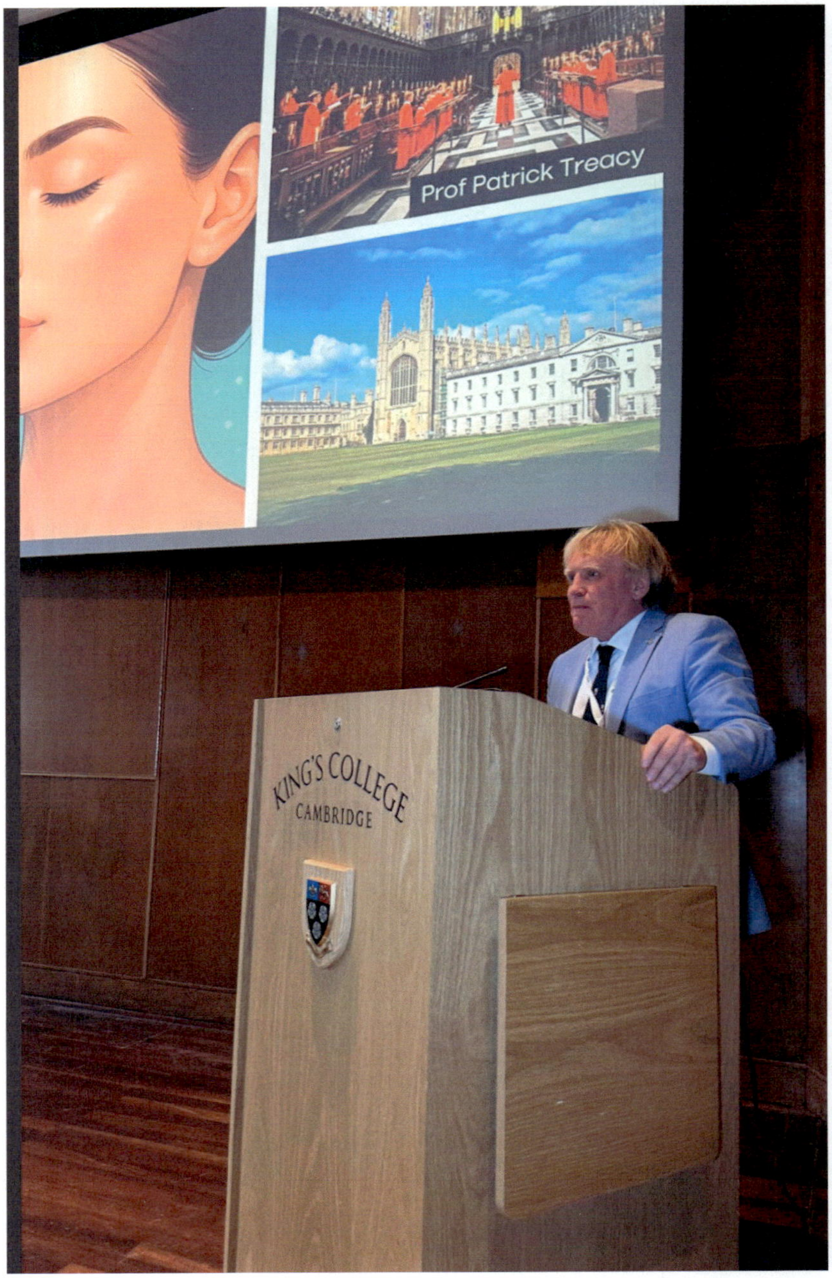

Prof Patrick Treacy lectures on Secretomes at the World Rejuvenation Conference (London)

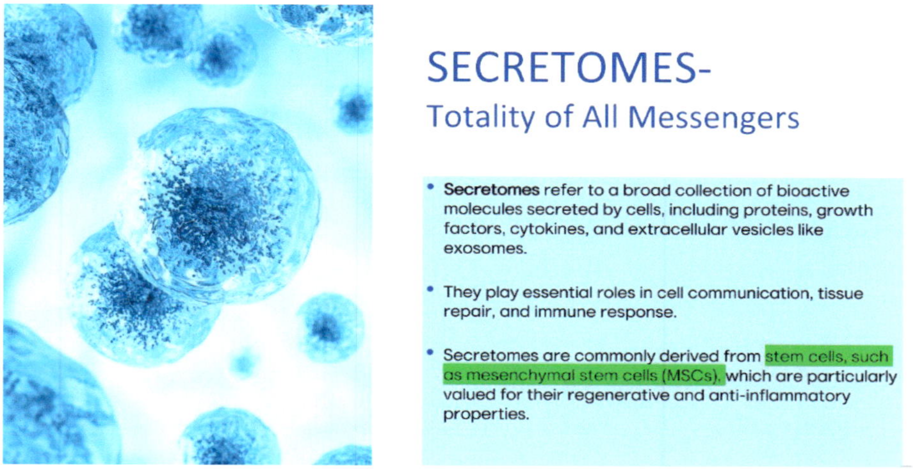

The Biological Roles of Secretomes

Secretomes are multifunctional, reflecting both the specific functions of their source cells and the influence of the local microenvironment. Secreted molecules bind to receptors on neighbouring or distant cells, coordinating processes such as **angiogenesis, tissue remodelling, and immune regulation**. In regenerative medicine, **MSCs' secretomes** are particularly valued for their ability to promote angiogenesis, accelerate tissue repair, and exert anti-inflammatory effects, making them ideal for applications in **wound healing and aesthetic rejuvenation**. By modulating immune cell behaviour, secretomes enhance tissue integration in grafts and implants, reducing inflammation and supporting healing. However, in pathological conditions such as **cancer or autoimmune disorders**, aberrant secretome profiles can exacerbate disease, driving metastasis or immune evasion, underscoring the need for precise therapeutic targeting.

The **MSC secretome**, enriched with cytokines, exosomes, and growth factors, plays a pivotal role in **modulating epithelial–mesenchymal transition (EMT)** and promoting **mesenchymal-to-epithelial transition (MET)**. This stabilises epithelial integrity and minimises scarring in burns and vascular occlusion recovery. Its regenerative functions are amplified by **RLT's ATP-boosting effects**, which enhance growth factor production, and by **PRP**, which stimulates fibroblast and keratinocyte activity. This synergy supports a robust **extracellular matrix (ECM)**, fostering re-epithelialisation and tissue homeostasis. Anti-inflammatory cytokines, such as **IL-10**, work alongside RLT's modulation of NF-κB activity to prevent excessive inflammation, ensuring an epithelial-friendly microenvironment conducive to MET and reducing fibrotic complications.

Secretome-Based Therapies in Regenerative Medicine

Secretome-based therapies are emerging as a powerful alternative to cell-based treatments, offering advantages in **safety, scalability, and consistency**. By delivering bioactive molecules such as **exosomes and growth factors**, rather than transplanting cells, these therapies circumvent challenges associated with cell survival, immune compatibility, and engraftment. In **aesthetic medicine**, secretome components—including exosome-rich formulations used since 2012—

support **skin rejuvenation, hair growth, and wound healing**, as demonstrated in the PLUS Technique. Beyond aesthetics, secretomes hold potential in **diagnostics**, where alterations in secretome profiles serve as biomarkers for disease progression, such as tumour metastasis, and in **drug development**, where identifying key secretome factors allows for targeted regenerative and anti-inflammatory therapies.

In the **revised PLUS Technique**, MSC secretomes' regenerative functions are further enhanced by **RLT** and **PRP**, creating a synergistic environment that supports MET while mitigating excessive EMT. This stabilises epithelial integrity and minimises fibrosis. Cytokines like **IL-10** and exosomes complement RLT's anti-inflammatory properties, reducing chronic inflammation and fostering an epithelial-friendly microenvironment. This approach accelerates **re-epithelialisation**, promotes tissue homeostasis, and is particularly effective in **burn treatment** and **post-vascular occlusion recovery**, where it restores tissue perfusion. The treatment protocol involves applying **PRP/MSC secretome mixtures** topically or intradermally, followed by RLT, with aftercare including additional RLT sessions and protective measures, such as wound dressings, to optimise healing.

Future Directions

Looking forward, secretome-based therapies are poised for significant advancements as of June 2025. Efforts are underway to **standardise isolation, characterisation, and quantification methods**, ensuring reproducible therapeutic quality. Personalized medicine is gaining traction, as understanding how secretomes adapt to specific microenvironments and genetic backgrounds may enable tailored therapies, enhancing efficacy in both aesthetic and clinical contexts. **Combination therapies**, integrating secretomes with **gene editing (e.g., CRISPR/Cas9), biomaterial scaffolds, or conventional cell therapies**, promise to maximise tissue repair synergy and drive innovations in tissue engineering and organ regeneration.

The PLUS Technique exemplifies this potential, demonstrating how **secretome-driven approaches**, combined with PRP and RLT, can transform regenerative aesthetics. It provides a framework for future therapies that address complex medical challenges, from **wound care to organ repair**, by leveraging synergistic, biologically-driven healing strategies.

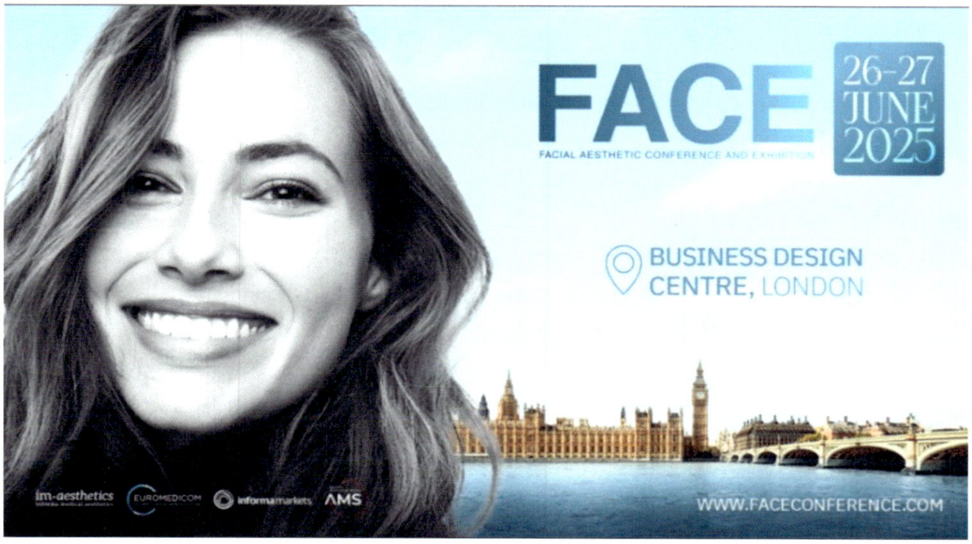

Prof Patrick Treacy lectures on Secretomes at FACE London 2025

Secretomes, the dynamic collection of molecules secreted by cells—including proteins, peptides, extracellular vesicles such as exosomes, lipid mediators, and other bioactive factors—play a central role in **intercellular communication and tissue regeneration**, making them a cornerstone of regenerative aesthetic protocols like the **PLUS Technique**. They contain **growth factors** such as Vascular Endothelial Growth Factor (VEGF) and Transforming Growth Factor Beta (TGF-β), **cytokines** including IL-6 and TNF-α, and **exosomes** carrying mRNAs and microRNAs. Together, these components orchestrate complex biological processes such as **wound healing, immune modulation, and tissue repair**.

In the PLUS Technique—which combines **Platelet-Rich Plasma (PRP), Mesenchymal Stem Cells (MSCs), and red-light therapy (RLT)** to treat skin injuries, burns, and post-vascular occlusion damage—the **MSC-derived secretome** plays a pivotal role by enhancing **epidermal regeneration, stimulating collagen synthesis, and modulating inflammation**. This activity synergises with PRP's growth factors and RLT's cellular stimulation to produce **rapid, natural, and durable regenerative outcomes**, supporting both functional recovery and aesthetic improvement.

Q 23 – How are Secretomes used in aesthetic medicine?

The applications of secretomes in **aesthetic medicine** are diverse, providing innovative solutions for **skin rejuvenation, hair restoration, and advanced wound care**, while offering a **safer, cell-free alternative** to traditional cell-based therapies. In **skin rejuvenation**, secretome-rich formulations—often containing growth factors and exosomes—are applied topically following **microneedling or laser treatments**, or administered via direct intradermal injection. These therapies **stimulate collagen synthesis, modulate inflammation, and enhance cellular turnover**, accelerating recovery, minimizing downtime, and producing **smoother, healthier skin with improved texture and reduced scarring**.

In **hair restoration**, secretome injections into the scalp **reactivate dormant hair follicles, promote new hair growth, and improve hair density and thickness** by optimizing the scalp microenvironment through enhanced **angiogenesis and nutrient delivery**. The **PLUS Technique** harnesses these regenerative properties by combining **MSC-derived secretomes, PRP growth factors, and the ATP-boosting effects of red-light therapy (RLT)**. This synergy **amplifies collagen remodeling and epithelial repair**, particularly in complex or high-risk cases such as **burns or post-vascular occlusion injuries**, supporting rapid, natural, and durable tissue regeneration.

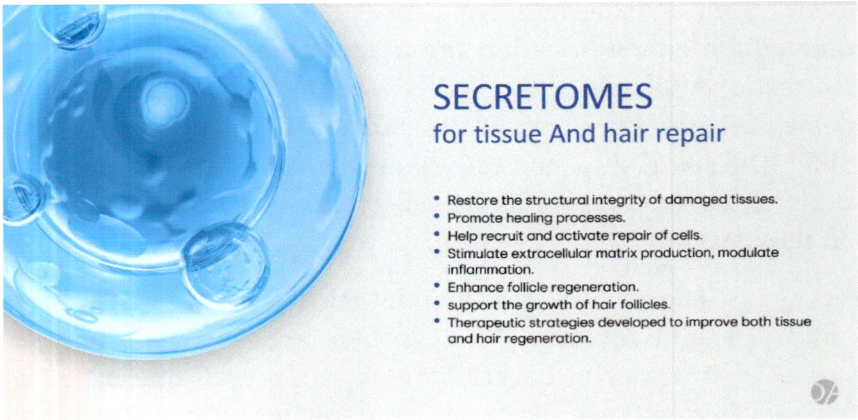

Secretomes, as **cell-free alternatives to stem cell transplantation**, reduce immunogenic risks and simplify regulatory considerations, making them a **scalable and safe option for aesthetic applications**. By delivering **bioactive molecules rather than live cells**, secretomes bypass challenges associated with cell survival, engraftment, and immune compatibility, enhancing therapeutic efficacy. They are often combined with complementary modalities such as **PRP, radiofrequency, or laser therapies** in protocols like the **PLUS Technique**, optimizing regenerative outcomes through **synergistic cellular crosstalk**.

For example, **MSC-derived secretomes** support **mesenchymal-to-epithelial transition (MET)**, stabilizing epithelial integrity and minimizing excessive **epithelial–mesenchymal transition (EMT)-driven fibrosis**, while **red-light therapy (RLT)** enhances these effects by boosting growth factor production and reducing inflammation. The **applications of secretomes in aesthetic**

medicine are diverse, including **skin rejuvenation, hair restoration, and advanced wound care**, offering a safer, cell-free alternative to traditional stem cell therapies.

In **skin rejuvenation**, secretome-rich formulations containing growth factors and exosomes are applied **topically after microneedling or laser treatments** or injected intradermally. These treatments **stimulate collagen synthesis, modulate inflammation, and enhance cellular turnover**, accelerating recovery, minimizing downtime, and improving skin texture while reducing scarring. For **hair restoration**, secretome injections into the scalp **reactivate dormant follicles, promote hair growth, and improve hair density and thickness** by optimizing the scalp microenvironment through **angiogenesis and nutrient delivery**.

The **PLUS Technique leverages these regenerative properties** by combining **MSC-derived secretomes, PRP growth factors, and RLT's ATP-enhancing effects**, amplifying collagen remodeling and epithelial repair, particularly in challenging cases such as **burns or vascular occlusions**. The treatment protocol involves applying **PRP/MSC secretome mixtures topically or intradermally**, followed by **633 nm RLT**, with aftercare including additional RLT sessions and protective measures such as **wound dressings or sun avoidance** to optimize healing.

The **efficacy of secretome-based therapies** depends on the source and processing of the secretome—typically derived from **MSCs or fibroblasts**—with consistent purity and stability being critical for reproducible outcomes. **Standardized isolation and quality control methods** are essential, as variations in cell type or processing can affect therapeutic results.

Looking forward, **secretome-based therapies are poised for significant advancements** as of June 2025. Efforts to **standardize and characterize secretomes** aim to ensure consistent therapeutic quality, while understanding how secretomes adapt to **specific microenvironments and genetic backgrounds** could enable **personalized treatments**. **Combining secretomes with biomaterials, gene editing (e.g., CRISPR/Cas9), or other regenerative modalities** promises to enhance tissue repair synergy, as exemplified by the PLUS Technique. These advancements position secretomes as a **cornerstone of regenerative aesthetics**, with applications extending to **advanced wound care** and potentially transforming **clinical practice in both aesthetic and medical contexts**.

Beyond aesthetic medicine, secretomes hold promise in **diagnostics and drug development**. Alterations in secretome profiles can serve as **biomarkers for disease progression**, identifying factors that drive **tumor metastasis or immune evasion**, enabling early diagnosis and targeted interventions. In **drug discovery**, key secretome components that modulate cellular pathways are being explored for **regenerative and anti-inflammatory therapies**, expanding their clinical potential.

In summary, the PLUS Technique exemplifies the **therapeutic power of secretomes**, where MSC-derived factors, PRP, and RLT synergistically **support MET, stabilize epithelial integrity, reduce EMT-driven fibrosis, enhance collagen and elastin deposition, and accelerate re-epithelialization**, delivering **natural, durable, and safe regenerative outcomes** in aesthetic and clinical applications.

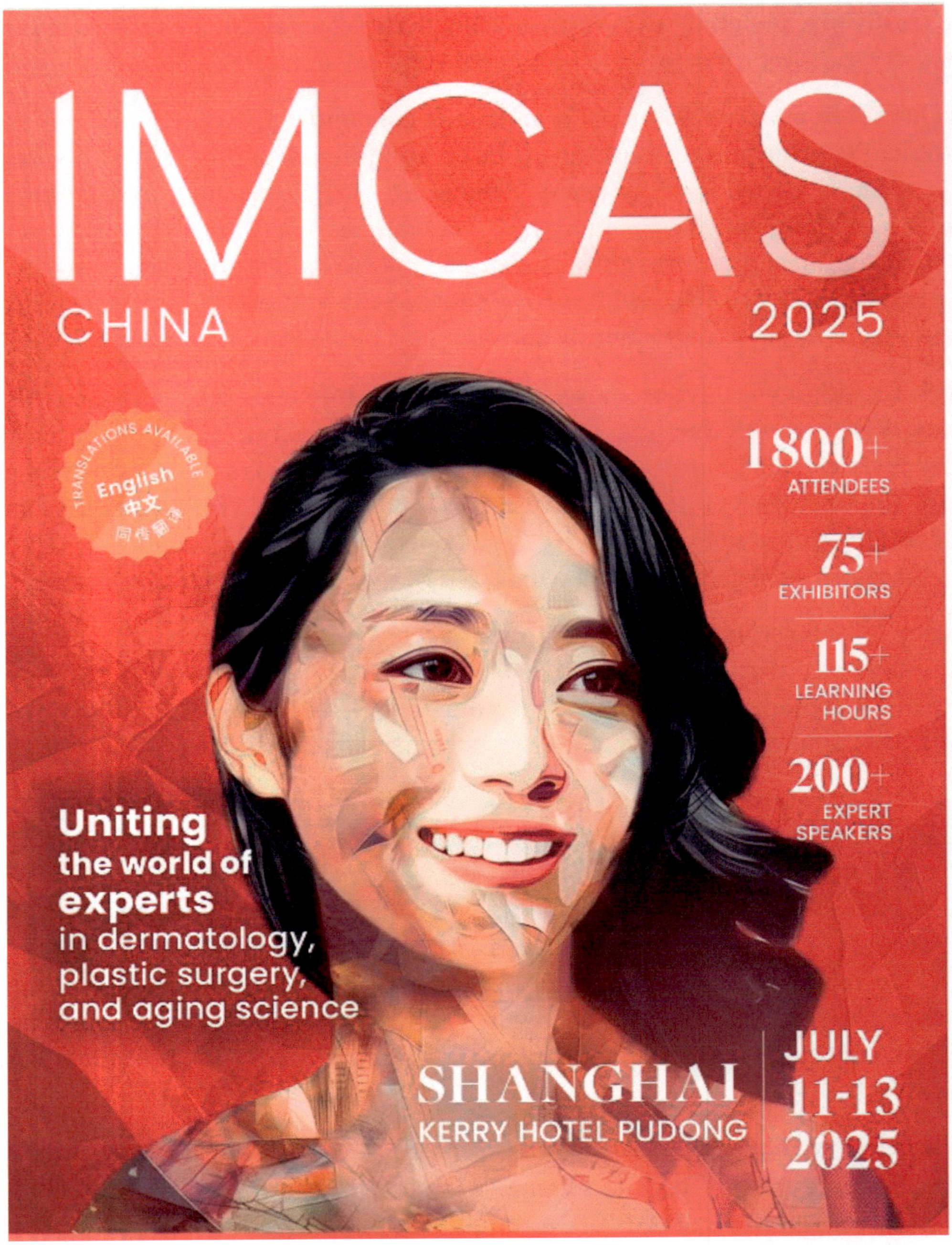

Prof Patrick Treacy lectures in Shanghai China on Secretomes

Beyond aesthetics, **secretomes hold considerable promise in diagnostics and drug development**. Changes in secretome profiles can serve as **biomarkers for disease progression**, enabling the identification of factors that drive **tumor metastasis or immune evasion** in cancer, facilitating **early diagnosis and targeted interventions**. In **drug discovery**, specific secretome components that modulate cellular pathways are being investigated for **regenerative and anti-inflammatory therapies**, expanding their clinical potential.

The **efficacy of secretome-based therapies** depends critically on the **cell source**—typically **MSCs or fibroblasts**—as well as the **purity and stability** of secreted factors, making **rigorous quality control essential**. In the **PLUS Technique**, the treatment protocol involves **topical or intradermal application of PRP/MSC secretome mixtures**, followed by **red-light therapy (RLT)**, with aftercare including additional RLT sessions and protective measures such as **wound dressings**. This approach ensures **optimized healing outcomes**, demonstrating the practical utility of secretomes in both aesthetic and clinical contexts.

Regulatory oversight is crucial as secretome-based therapies continue to advance. Current and evolving guidelines, including those referenced by the **FDA as of June 2025**, emphasize the need for **robust evidence validating secretome products**, addressing concerns related to **consistency, safety, and potential risks**. Future directions include the **standardization of isolation, quantification, and characterization methods** to ensure **therapeutic quality and reproducibility**.

Personalized medicine is also emerging as a key frontier, with insights into how secretomes respond to **specific microenvironments and genetic backgrounds** enabling the development of **tailored therapies**. Moreover, combining secretomes with **biomaterials, gene editing technologies such as CRISPR/Cas9, or other regenerative modalities** promises to **enhance tissue repair synergy**, as exemplified in the PLUS Technique model.

Collectively, these advancements position secretomes as a **dynamic and high-impact area of biomedical research**, with transformative potential across **regenerative medicine, oncology, and beyond**, offering the possibility of **redefining clinical practice and improving patient outcomes**.

Q 24 – How Do Secretomes or Exosomes work in Hair Growth?

In **hair restoration**, secretomes and exosomes **reactivate dormant hair follicles** by extending the **anagen (growth) phase** of the hair cycle. They deliver **microRNAs and growth factors** that stimulate **follicle stem cells** to re-enter a productive growth cycle, resulting in **thicker, stronger hair strands**. Anti-inflammatory cytokines within exosomes, such as **IL-10**, reduce chronic scalp inflammation, which can otherwise compromise follicle health, thereby creating a **favorable environment for hair growth**. Additionally, **VEGF and other angiogenic factors** enhance **vascularization**, improving blood flow to ensure follicles receive adequate **nutrients and oxygen**, while secreted proteins strengthen the **extracellular matrix (ECM)**, providing a supportive tissue framework around the follicles.

These regenerative functions are **further amplified in the PLUS Technique**, where **MSC-derived secretomes** synergize with **PRP's growth factors** and **RLT's ATP-boosting effects**, optimizing **cellular metabolism, tissue repair, and follicle regeneration**. This integrated approach aligns with the technique's broader applications in **skin rejuvenation and wound healing**.

Delivery methods for secretomes and exosomes are tailored to maximize therapeutic efficacy. **Targeted scalp injections** deliver high concentrations of regenerative factors directly to areas of thinning hair, while **topical application combined with microneedling** creates microchannels in the scalp, enhancing penetration and triggering a **regenerative response**. The PLUS Technique integrates both approaches, combining **PRP/MSC secretome mixtures** with **RLT**, while aftercare includes additional RLT sessions and protective measures such as **scalp care** to optimize recovery.

Combination therapies further amplify regenerative effects. Pairing secretomes with **PRP** or **low-level laser therapy (LLLT)** promotes **enhanced blood flow, follicle activation, and tissue rejuvenation**, exemplifying the PLUS Technique's **holistic, synergistic approach** to hair restoration.

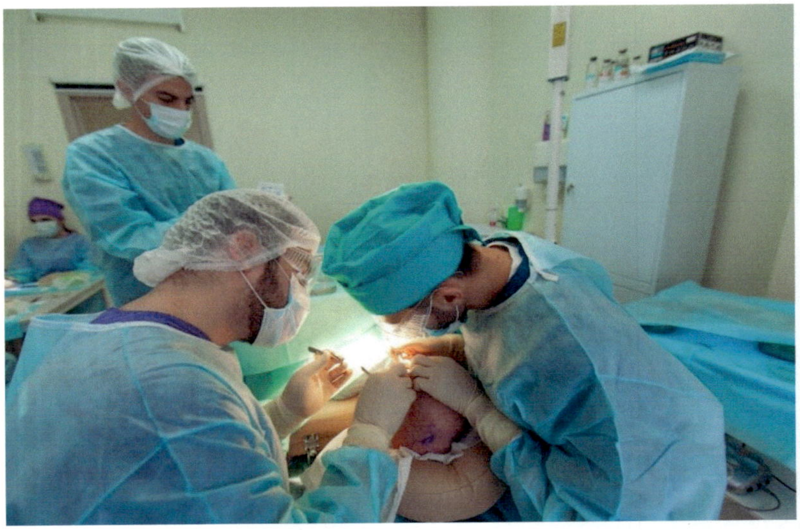

The efficacy of **secretome- and exosome-based therapies** depends on the **quality, source, and processing** of the bioactive substances, typically derived from **mesenchymal stem cells (MSCs), adipose-derived stem cells, or fibroblasts**. Maintaining **consistent purity, stability, and standardized processing protocols** is critical to ensure reproducible therapeutic outcomes, as variations in cell source or isolation methods can significantly affect efficacy. Regulatory oversight is evolving, with ongoing research focused on **standardizing isolation, storage, and delivery techniques** to minimize variability and ensure safety. While short-term studies report minimal adverse effects, **long-term data and larger clinical trials** are needed to fully validate efficacy, particularly in **hair restoration applications**. **Patient-specific factors**, such as age, pattern of hair loss, underlying health, and adherence to supportive treatments like nutrition and scalp care, also influence outcomes, highlighting the need for **personalized approaches**.

As of **June 2025**, the future of secretome- and exosome-based therapies in **hair restoration** is highly promising. Efforts to **standardize characterization and isolation methods** are helping to ensure consistent therapeutic quality. **Personalized medicine** is gaining momentum, as understanding how secretomes adapt to individual **microenvironments and genetic profiles** could enable tailored treatments. Combining secretomes with **biomaterials, gene editing, or complementary regenerative modalities**, as exemplified by the **PLUS Technique's integration of PRP and RLT**, has the potential to enhance outcomes in **tissue engineering and hair restoration**. These advancements position secretomes and exosomes as a **cornerstone of regenerative aesthetics**, with the capacity to transform clinical practice in hair restoration and beyond, offering patients **natural, effective, and durable rejuvenation**.

In summary: Secretomes and exosomes support hair restoration by delivering **potent signaling molecules** that **promote follicle health, reduce inflammation, and optimize the scalp microenvironment**. While current research and clinical applications are promising, further studies are essential to **refine protocols, standardize formulations, and determine the most effective strategies** for harnessing these regenerative therapies to achieve **consistent, long-term hair regrowth**.

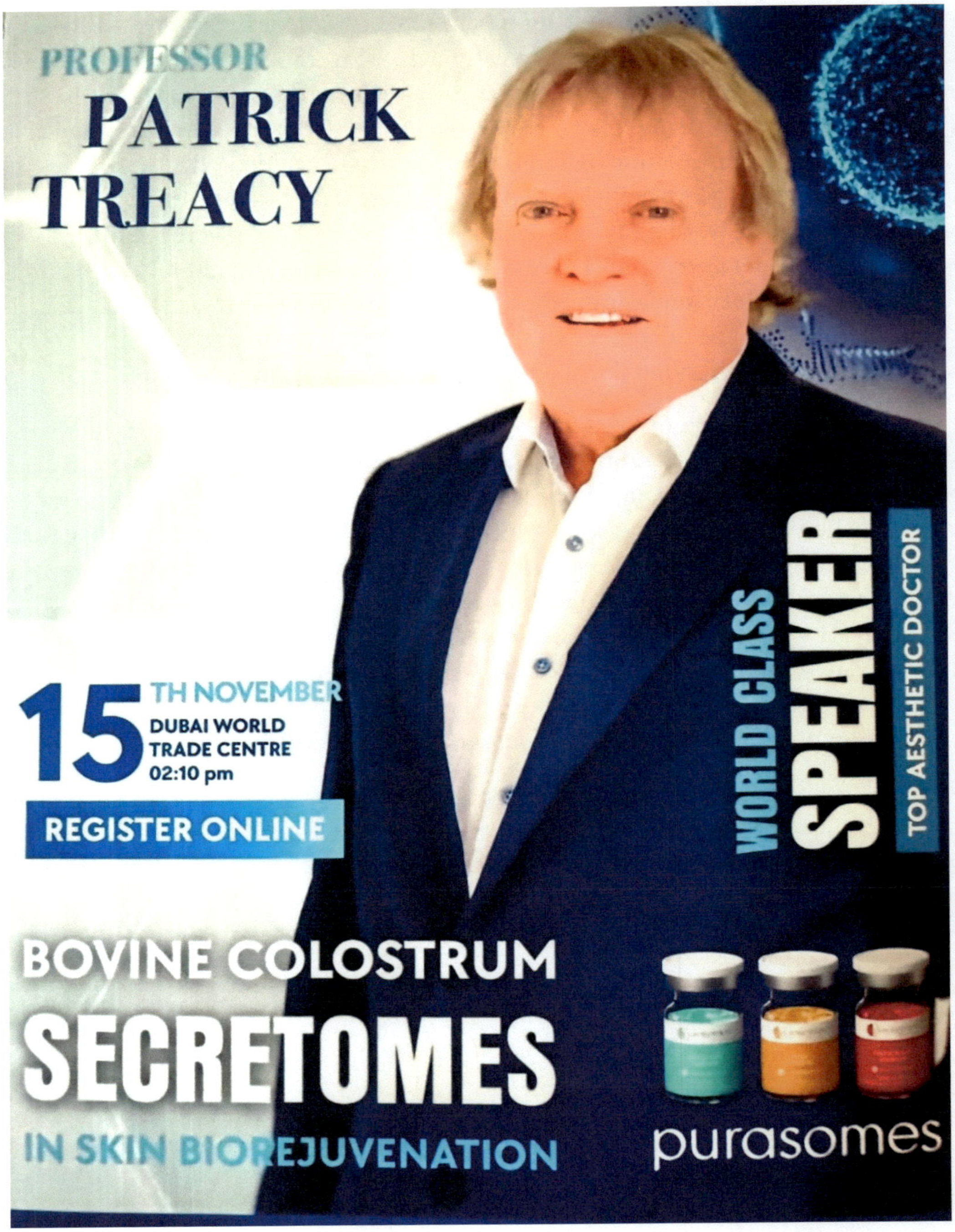

Prof Patrick Treacy lecturing in Dubai World Trade Centre (2024) about the use of Bovine Colostrum Secretomes in hair growth

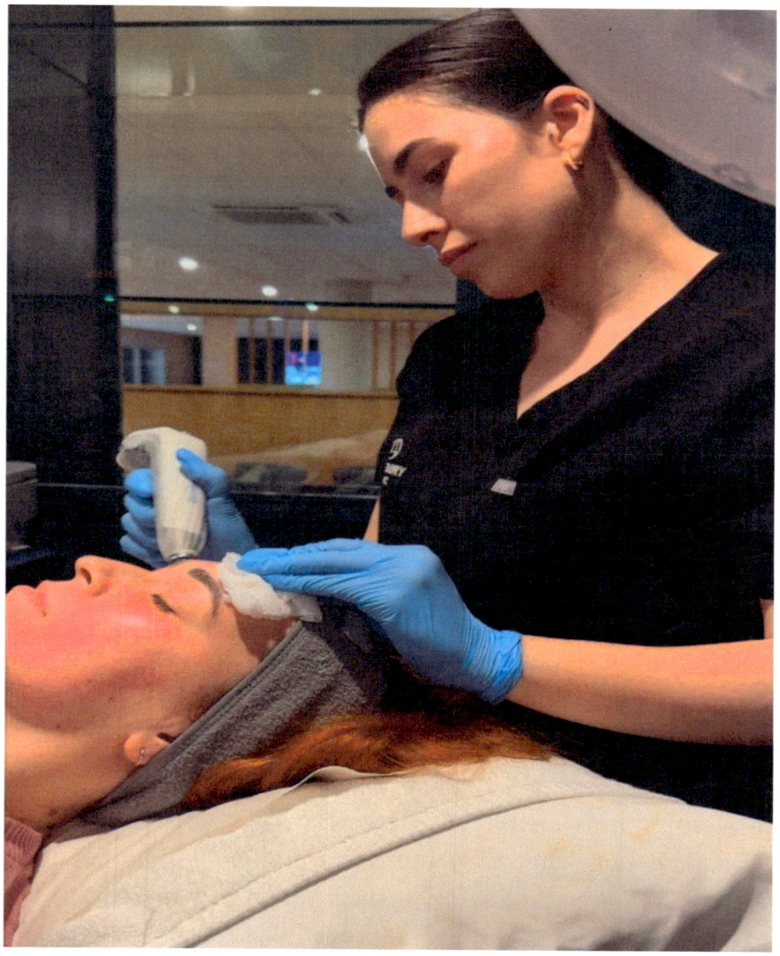

Patient receiving exosomes for restoration of hair growth at Ailesbury Dublin

Exosomes in Hair Restoration

Exosomes are emerging as a promising therapy for **hair growth restoration**, particularly in patients with **androgenetic alopecia (AGA)**—commonly referred to as male or female pattern baldness—and **alopecia areata**. These small **extracellular vesicles**, derived from stem cells such as **mesenchymal stem cells (MSCs)** or **dermal papilla cells (DPCs)**, contain **growth factors, proteins, lipids, and nucleic acids** that facilitate **cell-to-cell communication** and **tissue regeneration**.

Mechanisms and Benefits

Exosomes are believed to stimulate hair follicles through the delivery of bioactive molecules that:

- **Activate Dormant Follicles:** Encourage follicles in the resting (telogen) phase to enter the growth (anagen) phase, potentially reversing follicle miniaturization seen in androgenetic alopecia.
- **Promote Angiogenesis:** Growth factors such as **Vascular Endothelial Growth Factor (VEGF)** enhance scalp blood flow, supplying follicles with essential nutrients and oxygen.

- **Reduce Inflammation:** Anti-inflammatory cytokines (e.g., **IL-10**) mitigate scalp inflammation, which is associated with alopecia areata and follicle damage.
- **Enhance Follicle Health:** Proteins and microRNAs (e.g., **miR-21, miR-29a**) protect follicles from damage, improving hair thickness and quality.

Clinical Evidence

- A **retrospective study** in South Korea involving 39 patients with alopecia treated with **adipose-derived MSC exosomes (ADSC-Exos)** over 12 weeks reported significant improvements in **hair density and thickness**, marking one of the few human trials to date.
- **Preclinical studies** in mice demonstrated that exosomes from ADSCs and DPCs can **accelerate the anagen phase, increase follicle proliferation, and delay catagen onset**, suggesting potential efficacy.
- A **prospective study** of 30 male patients (aged 22–65) using **foreskin-derived MSC exosomes** reported reduced hair loss and improved growth by weeks 4 and 12; however, the lack of a control group limits the study's conclusiveness.

Treatment Approaches

Exosomes are most commonly **injected directly into the scalp**, often combined with **microneedling** to enhance penetration. Some therapies use **microneedle patches or topical serums** for a less invasive delivery. Exosomes are frequently paired with **Platelet-Rich Plasma (PRP)** or **red-light therapy (RLT)** to amplify regenerative effects.

Exosomes are generally considered **safe**, with minimal adverse effects reported, such as mild redness or swelling at injection sites. Being derived from **autologous or ethically sourced donor cells**, they carry a low risk of immune rejection. However, the **FDA has issued warnings** regarding unregulated exosome products due to potential contamination or inconsistent quality, highlighting the importance of **standardized manufacturing**.

Limitations

- Most evidence is derived from **preclinical studies or small human trials**; large, controlled clinical trials are limited.
- Efficacy depends on **exosome source, isolation methods (e.g., ultracentrifugation), and dosage**, which are not yet standardized.
- Treatments are **expensive** (often starting at £395 per session), with maintenance required every 6–12 months.
- Effects typically last 6–12 months, unlike hair transplants, which provide more permanent results.
- Best suited for **early-stage hair loss** (e.g., thinning or receding hairlines) rather than advanced baldness with fully atrophied follicles.

- May benefit patients unresponsive to conventional therapies like **minoxidil or finasteride**, or those seeking non-surgical alternatives.
- Not recommended for **severe scarring alopecia**, as exosomes cannot regenerate fully lost follicles.

CosmeRNA: An Innovative Anti-Hair Loss Therapy

CosmeRNA is an advanced anti-hair loss tonic developed by the South Korean company **Bioneer**, targeting **androgenetic alopecia (AGA)**, the most common form of hair loss in men and women. As of **30 June 2025**, it is gaining attention as a **non-hormonal alternative** to traditional treatments like minoxidil and finasteride.

Mechanism of Action

CosmeRNA uses **proprietary small interfering RNA (siRNA) technology**, specifically **Self-Assembled Micelle Inhibitory RNA (SAMiRNA)**, branded as **SAMiRNA-AR68 (AR68)**. It targets **androgen receptor (AR) mRNA** within hair follicles, reducing AR protein expression. Since **dihydrotestosterone (DHT)** drives follicle miniaturization and hair thinning in AGA, suppressing AR locally aims to **extend the anagen phase** and reduce hair loss without systemic hormonal side effects, such as those associated with finasteride (e.g., decreased libido or erectile dysfunction).

Delivery and Safety

The siRNA is delivered in **micellar form (<100 nm)**, designed for **efficient follicular penetration** when massaged into the scalp. This formulation **avoids immune activation** common with conventional siRNA, enhancing safety

Q 25 – Tell me about what happens during Cellular ageing.

Cellular aging is a complex biological process that progressively reduces the **functionality of cells, tissues, and organs**. In the skin, aging is particularly evident through changes in **fibroblast activity, growth factor secretion, extracellular matrix (ECM) composition, and the inflammatory milieu**. Key factors contributing to these age-related alterations include:

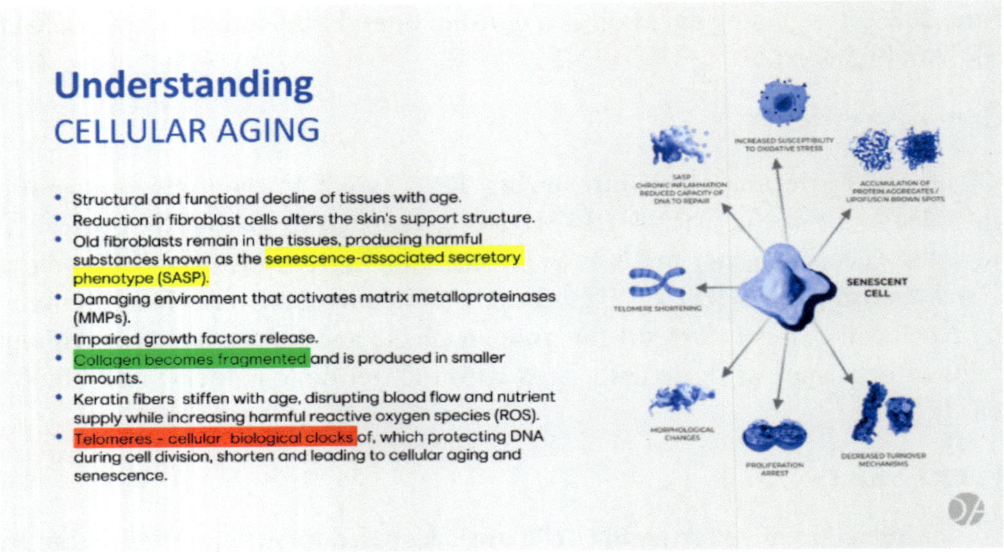

Aging profoundly affects skin structure and function, driven by declining fibroblast activity, impaired growth factor signaling, tissue thinning, compromised keratinocyte function, and oxidative stress from reactive oxygen species (ROS). The PLUS Technique, an advanced evolution of the Dublin Lift, addresses these age-related changes through the **synergistic integration of Platelet-Rich Plasma (PRP), Mesenchymal Stem Cells (MSCs), and red-light therapy (RLT)**.

With age, fibroblasts—the primary cells responsible for synthesizing collagen, elastin, and other extracellular matrix (ECM) components—exhibit reduced proliferation and diminished functional capacity. This decline slows wound healing, thins the dermis, and reduces skin elasticity, contributing to wrinkles, sagging, and other visible signs of aging due to compromised structural support. Simultaneously, the production and release of key growth factors, including Transforming Growth Factor Beta (TGF-β), Platelet-Derived Growth Factor (PDGF), and Fibroblast Growth Factor (FGF), decrease, while aged fibroblasts express fewer or less responsive growth factor receptors. These changes impair intercellular communication and limit tissue regeneration.

The PLUS Technique mitigates these deficits by combining PRP-derived growth factors with MSC-secreted bioactive molecules, including exosomes rich in VEGF and TGF-β. This combination **stimulates fibroblast proliferation, enhances collagen and elastin synthesis, and restores extracellular matrix integrity**, ultimately rejuvenating skin structure, improving elasticity, and promoting a more youthful appearance.

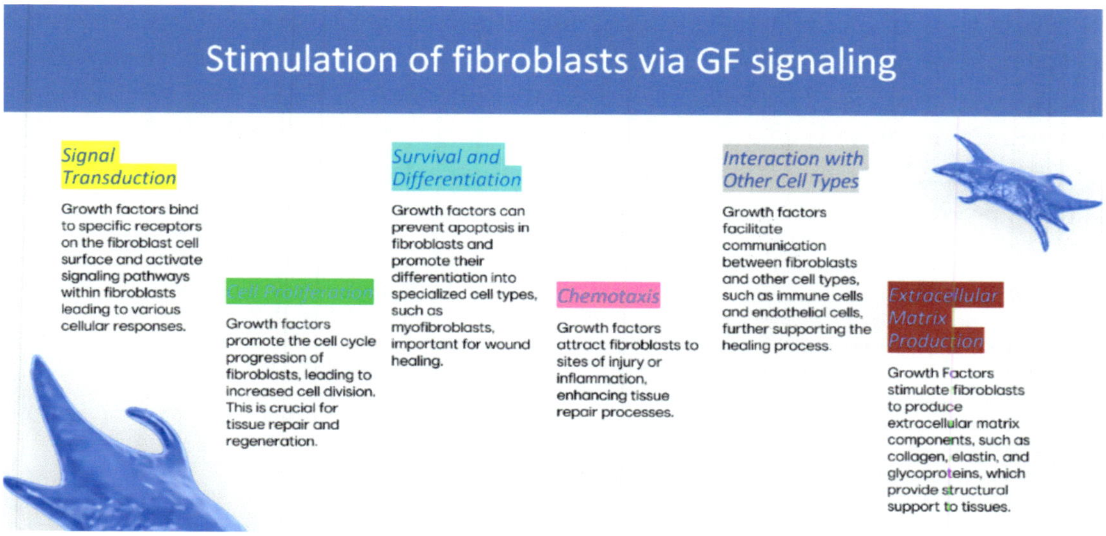

The decline in tissue integrity further accelerates aging. Reduced vascularisation, driven by diminished angiogenic signals such as Vascular Endothelial Growth Factor (VEGF), limits nutrient and oxygen delivery, slowing tissue renewal and compromising skin health. The epidermis, primarily composed of keratinocytes, also suffers: reduced cellular turnover weakens the skin's barrier function, increasing susceptibility to environmental stressors and resulting in drier, more fragile skin. Aging keratinocytes receive fewer rejuvenating signals from dysfunctional fibroblasts, disrupting cellular crosstalk and exacerbating skin deterioration.

Many fibroblasts enter a state of cellular senescence, ceasing division while remaining metabolically active. These senescent cells exhibit a **Senescence-Associated Secretory Phenotype (SASP)**, releasing pro-inflammatory cytokines, proteases, and growth factors that further disrupt tissue structure and propagate inflammation. The PLUS Technique mitigates these effects by leveraging MSC-derived secretomes, which contain anti-inflammatory cytokines such as IL-10, to modulate inflammation, promote **mesenchymal-to-epithelial transition (MET)**, stabilise epithelial integrity, and reduce fibrosis. Red-light therapy (RLT), typically delivered at ~633 nm, amplifies these effects by boosting ATP production, upregulating antioxidant enzymes like superoxide dismutase (SOD), and modulating NF-κB activity, creating an epithelial-friendly microenvironment conducive to tissue repair.

Oxidative stress from reactive oxygen species (ROS), including superoxide anions and hydrogen peroxide, accelerates cellular aging by damaging DNA, proteins, and lipids, particularly under environmental stressors such as UV exposure and pollution. Elevated ROS levels contribute to telomere shortening, fibroblast senescence, chronic inflammation, and impaired tissue repair. Aging cells also produce fewer endogenous antioxidants, such as SOD and glutathione, weakening their defense against oxidative damage.

In hair restoration, a major application of the PLUS Technique, chronic inflammation and oxidative stress can compromise follicle health. MSC-derived secretomes deliver key growth factors, including FGF, VEGF, and Insulin-Like Growth Factor (IGF), alongside microRNAs, to **extend the anagen (growth) phase, reactivate dormant follicles, and enhance vascularisation**. The protocol involves scalp injections or topical application of PRP/MSC secretome mixtures post-microneedling, followed by RLT, with aftercare incorporating additional RLT sessions to optimise outcomes. This integrated approach not only counteracts age-related decline in skin and hair but also promotes robust, multi-layered tissue regeneration.

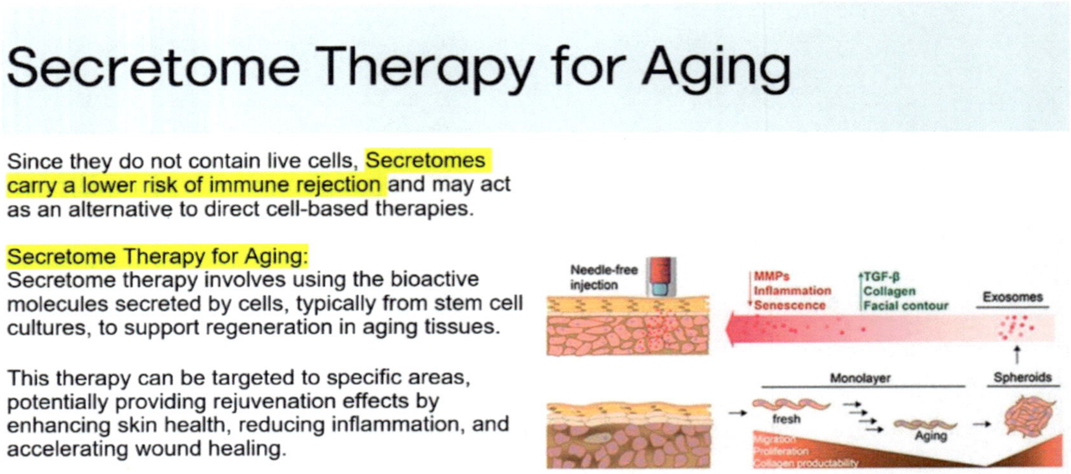

The PLUS Technique's integration of secretomes reflects current trends in regenerative medicine. Secretome-based therapies provide a **cell-free alternative to stem cell transplantation**, reducing immunogenic risks and simplifying regulatory requirements, as demonstrated in applications for skin rejuvenation and hair restoration. Efforts to **standardise secretome isolation, processing, and quality control** are ongoing to ensure consistent therapeutic efficacy, while personalised approaches that account for individual microenvironmental and genetic factors promise tailored, optimised treatments.

Combining secretomes with **biomaterials or gene-editing technologies** such as CRISPR/Cas9 has the potential to further enhance regenerative outcomes, building upon the PLUS Technique's synergistic integration of PRP, MSCs, and red-light therapy (RLT). Regulatory oversight continues to evolve, with guidelines focused on ensuring safety and efficacy and addressing challenges such as variability in secretome composition and processing. By counteracting age-related skin deterioration and promoting structured tissue repair, the PLUS Technique exemplifies the transformative potential of secretome-based therapies, establishing a foundation for **future innovations in both aesthetic and clinical regenerative applications**.

Q 26 – What is the SASP (Senescence-Associated Secretory Phenotype) molecule?

Cellular ageing profoundly impairs skin and hair health through reduced fibroblast function, compromised tissue integrity, diminished keratinocyte activity, and oxidative stress from reactive oxygen species (ROS). The **Senescence-Associated Secretory Phenotype (SASP)** further accelerates tissue decline by promoting chronic, low-grade inflammation. Fibroblasts, which are essential for synthesising collagen, elastin, and extracellular matrix (ECM) components, show reduced proliferation and efficiency with age. This is compounded by fewer or less responsive growth factor receptors, impairing regenerative signalling mediated by molecules such as **Transforming Growth Factor Beta (TGF-β), Platelet-Derived Growth Factor (PDGF), and Fibroblast Growth Factor (FGF)**. The resulting structural deficits manifest as a thinner dermis, wrinkles, and sagging.

Ageing also diminishes angiogenic signalling, including **Vascular Endothelial Growth Factor (VEGF)**, reducing vascularisation and limiting nutrient and oxygen delivery, thereby slowing tissue renewal. Keratinocytes, key to maintaining the skin's barrier function, exhibit reduced turnover, weakening the epidermal barrier and increasing susceptibility to environmental stressors. The disrupted crosstalk between keratinocytes and fibroblasts further accelerates skin deterioration.

Regenerative strategies—such as **Platelet-Rich Plasma (PRP), mesenchymal stem cells (MSCs), and red-light therapy (RLT)**—counteract these deficits by stimulating fibroblast activity and collagen synthesis. Dr. Treacy's 2021 modification of the PLUS Technique, incorporating **Purosomes** from DermaAroma (Italy), derived from bovine colostrum, enhances outcomes by delivering bioactive molecules including immunoglobulins and growth factors like **IGF-1 and TGF-β**, further supporting tissue repair and rejuvenation as of June 30, 2025.

SASP, a hallmark of cellular senescence, significantly contributes to tissue ageing. Senescent fibroblasts, although no longer dividing, remain metabolically active and secrete pro-inflammatory cytokines, chemokines, proteases (e.g., **matrix metalloproteinases**), and growth factors. These secretions fuel chronic inflammation—referred to as "inflammaging"—and degrade collagen and other ECM components, weakening tissue structure. SASP also exerts paracrine effects that induce senescence in neighbouring cells, amplifying a damaging cycle that promotes fibrosis and impairs tissue repair. In hair restoration, SASP-driven inflammation compromises follicle health, reducing hair density and thickness.

Oxidative stress from ROS, such as superoxide anions and hydrogen peroxide, is exacerbated by environmental factors like UV exposure and pollution. Elevated ROS levels accelerate ageing by damaging DNA, proteins, and lipids, contributing to telomere shortening and fibroblast senescence. Ageing cells produce fewer antioxidants, such as **superoxide dismutase (SOD)** and glutathione, weakening defence mechanisms and perpetuating inflammation.

Regenerative interventions, including **MSC-derived secretomes** and Purosomes, deliver anti-inflammatory cytokines such as **IL-10** to mitigate SASP-driven inflammation. RLT at approximately 633 nm complements these effects by upregulating antioxidant enzymes and modulating **NF-κB** activity, creating an epithelial-friendly microenvironment that promotes **mesenchymal-to-epithelial transition (MET)** and minimises excessive **epithelial–mesenchymal transition (EMT)-driven fibrosis**.

Q 27 – Tell me about the Reduction in Fibroblast Cells during ageing

Fibroblasts are specialized cells predominantly located in connective tissue, where they are essential for producing and maintaining the **extracellular matrix (ECM)**—a network of proteins such as collagen and elastin that provides structural support, elasticity, and a scaffold for cell proliferation and migration. Their activity is central to **wound healing, tissue repair, and overall skin and hair health**.

Fibroblasts act as the primary architects of connective tissue, synthesizing ECM components while secreting growth factors—including **Fibroblast Growth Factor (FGF), Transforming Growth Factor Beta (TGF-β), and Platelet-Derived Growth Factor (PDGF)**—to stimulate neighbouring cells and coordinate regenerative processes. In response to injury, activated fibroblasts migrate to the wound site, depositing new collagen and ECM to restore tissue integrity, making them indispensable for maintaining skin resilience and supporting hair follicle health.

However, **ageing significantly impairs fibroblast function**. Senescent fibroblasts exhibit reduced proliferative capacity, produce lower-quality collagen, and secrete fewer growth factors, resulting in thinner, less elastic skin, slower tissue repair, and visible signs of ageing such as wrinkles and sagging. Ageing fibroblasts also express fewer or less responsive growth factor receptors, disrupting regenerative signalling pathways.

Regenerative interventions—including **Platelet-Rich Plasma (PRP), mesenchymal stem cells (MSCs), and red-light therapy (RLT)**—counteract these deficits by stimulating fibroblast activity, enhancing collagen synthesis, and promoting ECM restoration. In 2021, Dr. Treacy modified the PLUS Technique to incorporate **Purosomes from DermaAroma, Italy**, derived from bovine colostrum. These vesicles are rich in immunoglobulins and growth factors such as **IGF-1 and TGF-β**, further enhancing fibroblast-mediated tissue repair and skin rejuvenation, with documented applications as of **June 30, 2025**.

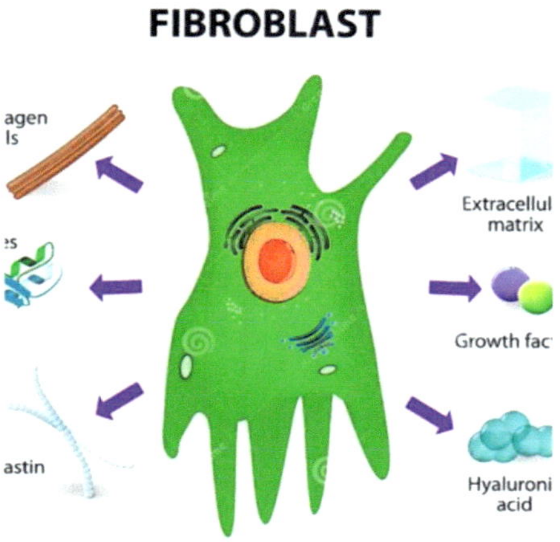

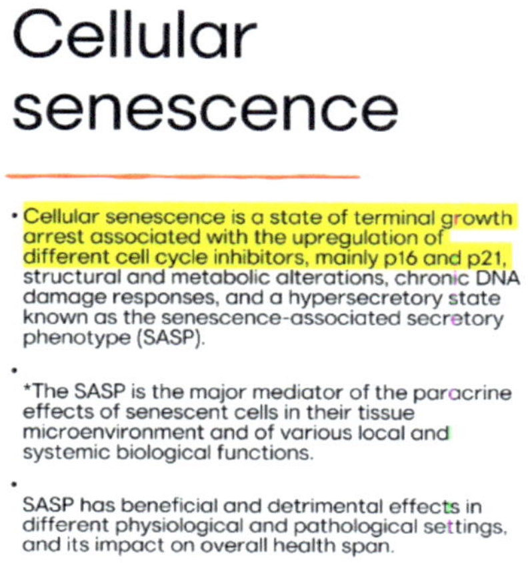

Cellular senescence exacerbates tissue ageing as fibroblasts enter a state of **cell cycle arrest** while remaining metabolically active. These senescent fibroblasts exhibit a **Senescence-Associated Secretory Phenotype (SASP)**, releasing pro-inflammatory cytokines, chemokines, proteases (e.g., matrix metalloproteinases), and growth factors. SASP contributes to **chronic, low-grade inflammation**, also known as *inflammaging*, which degrades collagen and ECM components, weakens tissue structure, and induces neighbouring cells to become senescent, amplifying a damaging cycle. In **hair restoration**, SASP-driven inflammation impairs follicle health, reducing hair density.

Oxidative stress from reactive oxygen species (ROS), including superoxide anions and hydrogen peroxide, is exacerbated by environmental factors such as UV exposure and pollution. ROS accelerate ageing by causing **DNA damage, protein and lipid oxidation, and telomere shortening**, further promoting fibroblast senescence. Ageing cells also produce fewer antioxidants, such as **superoxide dismutase (SOD)** and glutathione, weakening defence mechanisms against ROS.

Regenerative interventions mitigate these effects. **MSC-derived secretomes** and **Purosomes** deliver anti-inflammatory cytokines like **IL-10**, reducing SASP-driven inflammation, while **red-light therapy (RLT) at ~633 nm** enhances antioxidant enzyme activity and modulates **NF-κB** signalling, creating an epithelial-friendly microenvironment that promotes **mesenchymal-to-epithelial transition (MET)** and limits excessive **epithelial–mesenchymal transition (EMT)-driven fibrosis**.

In **aesthetic applications**—including skin rejuvenation and hair restoration—these regenerative strategies restore fibroblast function and counteract age-related decline. MSC secretomes and Purosomes provide growth factors such as **FGF, VEGF, and IGF-1**, along with microRNAs, to reactivate dormant hair follicles, extend the **anagen (growth) phase**, and enhance scalp vascularisation, improving hair density and thickness. For skin, these interventions stimulate collagen synthesis, reorganise the ECM, reduce wrinkles, and strengthen barrier function.

Treatment protocols typically involve topical or intradermal application of secretome-rich mixtures (sometimes including Purosomes) post-microneedling, followed by RLT, with aftercare including additional RLT sessions and protective measures such as scalp care or wound dressings to optimise outcomes. Regulatory oversight for secretome-based therapies, including bovine colostrum-derived Purosomes, is evolving to ensure **safety, consistency, and efficacy**, with ongoing efforts to standardise isolation and processing methods.

Future directions as of June 2025 include combining secretomes with **biomaterials, gene editing technologies (e.g., CRISPR/Cas9), senolytics to remove senescent cells, and antioxidant therapies** to mitigate ROS, positioning regenerative aesthetics as a transformative approach for counteracting age-related decline in skin and hair.

Summary:

- **Fibroblasts** are central to tissue growth, maintenance, and repair through ECM production and growth factor secretion.

- **Cellular ageing** in fibroblasts is characterised by reduced collagen synthesis, impaired regenerative capacity, and senescence, contributing to visible and functional tissue decline.
- **Regenerative strategies**—including antioxidants, secretome therapies, and senolytics—are being investigated to support fibroblast function, mitigate age-related degeneration, and improve skin and hair health.

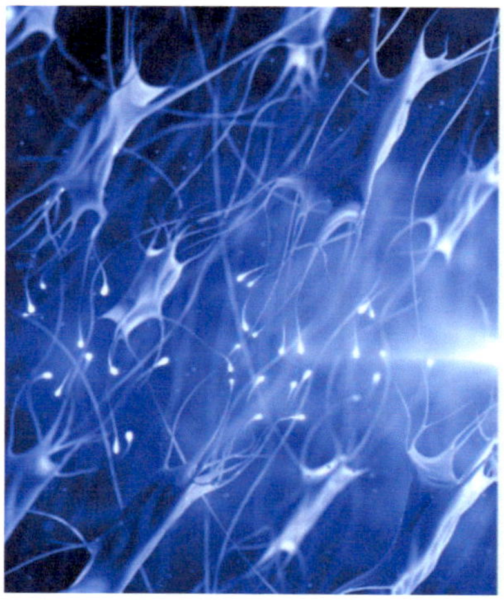

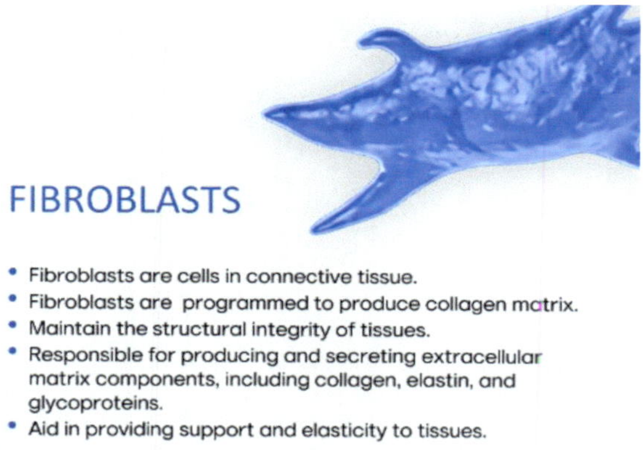

Fibroblasts are **key architects of connective tissues**, driving cell growth and tissue maintenance by secreting **extracellular matrix (ECM) components** and growth factors that provide structural support and coordinate the activity of surrounding cells. As fibroblasts **age or enter senescence**, their regenerative capacity declines, and they may actively contribute to tissue ageing by releasing **pro-inflammatory signals**. Consequently, strategies aimed at **preserving or restoring fibroblast function**—including antioxidant therapies, senolytics, and regenerative interventions—have become central to efforts to **slow or counteract age-related tissue decline**.

Q 28 – Tell me about Impaired Growth Factor Release during ageing

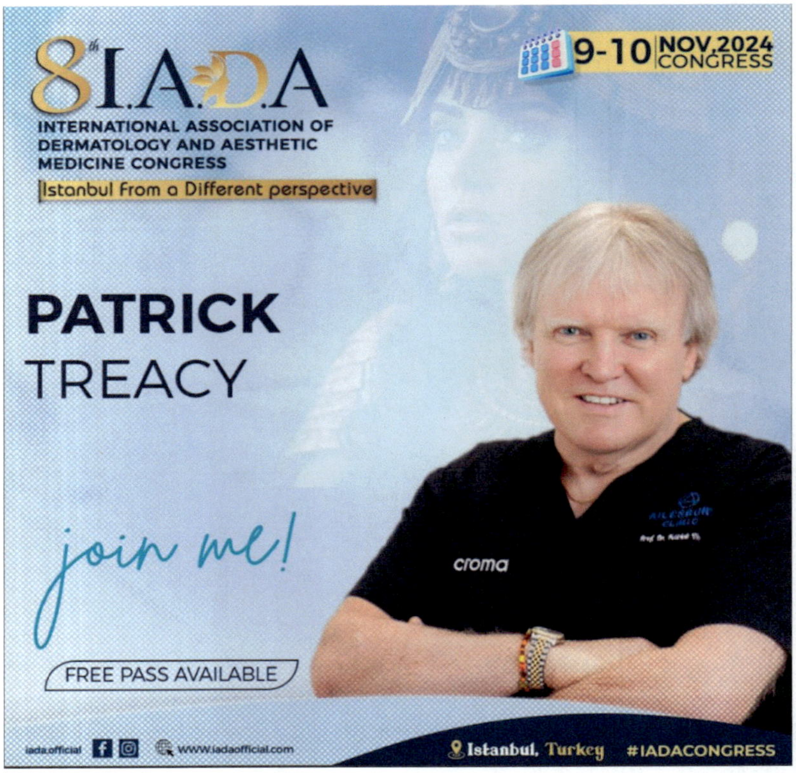

As the body ages, the decline in growth factor secretion by cells such as fibroblasts markedly impairs tissue maintenance and repair, contributing to visible signs of ageing, including wrinkles, thinning skin, and compromised hair follicle health. Regenerative aesthetic strategies address these challenges through interventions such as Platelet-Rich Plasma (PRP), mesenchymal stem cell (MSC)-derived secretomes, and red-light therapy (RLT). Fibroblasts exhibit reduced secretion of critical growth factors—Transforming Growth Factor Beta (TGF-β), Platelet-Derived Growth Factor (PDGF), and Fibroblast Growth Factors (FGFs)—which are essential for collagen synthesis, wound healing, and cell renewal. This decline, compounded by fewer or less responsive growth factor receptors, disrupts cell-to-cell communication, slowing tissue regeneration and weakening structural integrity in the skin and other tissues.

Cellular senescence exacerbates this decline, as senescent fibroblasts accumulate in ageing tissues and adopt a **Senescence-Associated Secretory Phenotype (SASP)**, releasing pro-inflammatory cytokines and proteases instead of reparative growth factors. This fuels chronic, low-grade inflammation—termed "inflammaging"—and impairs regenerative signalling. Regenerative approaches, enhanced by Dr. Treacy's 2021 modification to include **Purosomes from DermaAroma, Italy**, derived from bovine colostrum and rich in bioactive molecules like IGF-1,

TGF-β, and immunoglobulins, counteract these deficits by delivering growth factors and anti-inflammatory cytokines to restore tissue vitality, as of June 30, 2025.

Oxidative stress from reactive oxygen species (ROS), including superoxide anions and hydrogen peroxide, driven by environmental factors such as UV exposure and pollution, further impairs growth factor production by damaging DNA, proteins, and lipids, and contributing to telomere shortening. Ageing cells produce fewer antioxidants, such as superoxide dismutase (SOD) and glutathione, weakening ROS defences and accelerating fibroblast senescence, which amplifies SASP-driven inflammation and extracellular matrix (ECM) degradation.

In hair restoration, this impaired signalling reduces follicle health and hair density. Regenerative interventions using MSC secretomes and Purosomes deliver growth factors such as FGF, VEGF, and IGF-1, alongside microRNAs, to reactivate dormant follicles, extend the anagen (growth) phase, and enhance scalp vascularisation. For skin rejuvenation, these therapies stimulate collagen synthesis and epithelial repair, countering dermal thinning, weakened barrier function, and disrupted fibroblast–keratinocyte crosstalk. Treatment protocols typically involve **topical or intradermal application of secretome-rich mixtures**, including Purosomes, post-microneedling, followed by **RLT at 633 nm** to boost ATP production and upregulate antioxidant enzymes. Aftercare often includes additional RLT sessions and protective measures, such as scalp care or wound dressings, to optimise outcomes.

The implications of impaired growth factor release extend across aesthetic and regenerative medicine, driving research into strategies that restore or replace diminished regenerative signals. PRP, exosome therapy, and MSC-based approaches compensate for reduced growth factor levels, promoting collagen synthesis, angiogenesis, and tissue repair. Concurrently, RLT mitigates oxidative stress and inflammation, creating an epithelial-friendly microenvironment that supports **mesenchymal-to-epithelial transition (MET)** and limits excessive **epithelial–mesenchymal transition (EMT)**–driven fibrosis. Regulatory oversight for secretome-based therapies, including bovine colostrum-derived Purosomes, is evolving to ensure safety and efficacy, with ongoing efforts to standardise isolation and processing methods to reduce variability.

As of June 2025, future directions include **combining secretomes with biomaterials, gene editing (e.g., CRISPR/Cas9), senolytics to remove senescent cells, and antioxidant therapies to mitigate ROS**, further enhancing regenerative outcomes. These advancements position regenerative aesthetics as a transformative field for addressing age-related decline in skin and hair, offering innovative strategies to restore tissue function, counteract senescence, and slow the ageing process.

Q 29 – What Is Cellular Senescence?

Cellular senescence is a state in which cells permanently stop dividing while remaining metabolically active. Although commonly regarded as a hallmark of aging, senescence is a complex process that can have both beneficial and detrimental effects on the body. Below is an overview of the key advantages and potential drawbacks associated with cellular senescence.

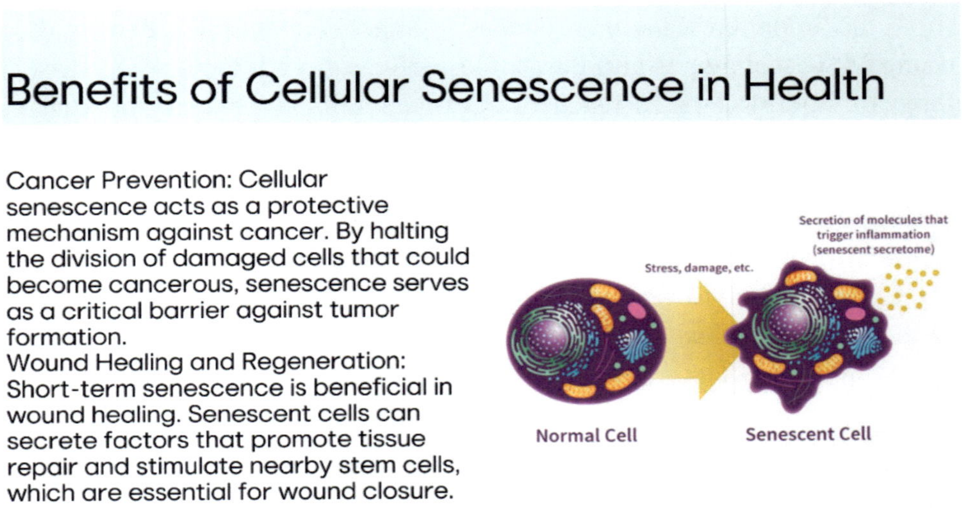

Cellular senescence, a state triggered by stressors such as DNA damage, oxidative stress, or telomere shortening, halts cell proliferation while maintaining metabolic activity. Senescent cells release a spectrum of signalling molecules that influence tissue health and ageing, presenting both benefits and challenges that regenerative aesthetic strategies aim to address.

As a protective mechanism, senescence prevents uncontrolled division of damaged cells, acting as a tumour-suppressive barrier by arresting the cell cycle in response to potential oncogenic signals. During wound healing and tissue remodelling, transiently senescent cells secrete growth factors and cytokines that recruit immune cells, clear cellular debris, and facilitate repair. In embryonic development, programmed senescence sculpts tissues by removing unnecessary cells.

However, chronic senescence contributes to age-related decline through the Senescence-Associated Secretory Phenotype (SASP). Senescent cells—including fibroblasts—release pro-inflammatory cytokines, chemokines, proteases (e.g., matrix metalloproteinases), and growth factors, driving “inflammaging.” This process degrades collagen and extracellular matrix (ECM) components, weakens tissue structure, and induces neighboring cells to become senescent via paracrine signalling. The result is amplified tissue dysfunction, reduced regenerative capacity, slower healing, and the development of age-associated conditions such as osteoarthritis and atherosclerosis, as well as visible signs of ageing like wrinkles and thinning skin, as of June 30, 2025.

The accumulation of senescent cells, exacerbated by declining immune clearance with age, impairs tissue turnover and metabolic homeostasis. Oxidative stress from reactive oxygen species (ROS), driven by environmental factors such as UV exposure and pollution, accelerates senescence by damaging DNA, proteins, and lipids while diminishing antioxidant defences, including superoxide dismutase (SOD) and glutathione. In hair restoration, SASP-driven inflammation and reduced growth factor secretion (e.g., TGF-β, PDGF, FGF) impair follicle health and decrease hair density.

Regenerative strategies counter these effects through interventions like Platelet-Rich Plasma (PRP), mesenchymal stem cell (MSC)-derived secretomes, and red-light therapy (RLT) at 633 nm. These approaches stimulate fibroblast activity, collagen synthesis, and angiogenesis while mitigating SASP-driven inflammation. Dr. Treacy's 2021 modification of the PLUS Technique incorporated Purosomes from DermaAroma, Italy—derived from bovine colostrum and rich in immunoglobulins, growth factors (e.g., IGF-1, TGF-β), and anti-inflammatory cytokines—to further enhance tissue repair and reduce inflammaging. These therapies promote mesenchymal-to-epithelial transition (MET), counter excessive epithelial–mesenchymal transition (EMT)-driven fibrosis, and restore skin and hair vitality by fostering an epithelial-friendly microenvironment.

Therapeutic approaches to balance senescence's beneficial and detrimental effects include senolytics, which selectively remove senescent cells, and senomorphics, which modulate SASP with anti-inflammatory compounds without eliminating cells. Regenerative therapies employing MSC secretomes, Purosomes, and RLT restore tissue function by delivering growth factors (e.g., FGF, VEGF, IGF-1) and anti-inflammatory cytokines (e.g., IL-10), while RLT upregulates antioxidant enzymes and modulates NF-κB activity to mitigate ROS and inflammaging.

Treatment protocols typically involve topical or intradermal application of secretome-rich mixtures, including Purosomes, post-microneedling, followed by RLT. Aftercare includes additional RLT sessions and protective measures, such as scalp care or wound dressings, to optimise outcomes in skin rejuvenation and hair restoration. Regulatory oversight for secretome-based therapies, including bovine colostrum-derived Purosomes, continues to evolve to ensure safety and efficacy, with standardisation efforts addressing variability.

As of June 2025, future directions include combining secretomes with biomaterials, gene editing (e.g., CRISPR/Cas9), and senolytics to enhance regenerative outcomes. These advancements position regenerative aesthetics as a transformative field for mitigating age-related decline and promoting healthy ageing.

Q 30 – What Does the SASP (Senescence-Associated Secretory Phenotype) molecule do?

Senescence-Associated Secretory Phenotype (SASP) refers to the distinct collection of pro-inflammatory and proteolytic factors—including cytokines, chemokines, growth factors, and proteases—secreted by senescent cells. Although these cells no longer divide, they remain metabolically active and profoundly influence their surrounding tissue environment through SASP.

The Dual Nature of SASP: Balancing Regeneration and Ageing in Aesthetic Medicine
Cellular senescence is a state of permanent cell-cycle arrest triggered by stressors such as DNA damage, telomere shortening, oxidative stress, or oncogenic signalling. Senescent cells remain metabolically active and secrete a complex array of molecules known as the Senescence-Associated Secretory Phenotype (SASP), which plays a dual role in tissue health and ageing, presenting both opportunities and challenges for regenerative aesthetic interventions.

SASP includes cytokines (e.g., IL-6, IL-8), chemokines, growth factors such as Transforming Growth Factor Beta (TGF-β), and proteases like matrix metalloproteinases (MMPs). These factors drive inflammation, recruit immune cells, remodel tissues, and degrade the extracellular matrix (ECM). In acute or controlled contexts, SASP is beneficial: it promotes tumour suppression by enabling immune clearance of potentially cancerous cells, aids wound healing through growth factor secretion and immune cell recruitment, and supports embryonic development by sculpting tissues.

However, chronic SASP contributes to "inflammaging," a persistent, low-grade inflammatory state that degrades collagen and ECM components, weakens tissue structure, and induces paracrine senescence in neighboring cells. This amplifies tissue dysfunction and accelerates ageing-related pathologies such as osteoporosis, atherosclerosis, and visible skin ageing, manifesting as wrinkles, thinning skin, and diminished elasticity.

The detrimental effects of chronic SASP are particularly relevant in aesthetic medicine. MMPs degrade ECM components, impairing skin integrity and hair follicle health, while paracrine senescence reduces tissue turnover, slowing repair and exacerbating visible signs of ageing. Oxidative stress from reactive oxygen species (ROS), driven by UV exposure and pollution, further amplifies SASP by damaging DNA, proteins, and lipids, while weakening endogenous antioxidant defences, including superoxide dismutase (SOD) and glutathione.

Regenerative strategies counter these effects by stimulating tissue repair and mitigating chronic inflammation. Interventions such as Platelet-Rich Plasma (PRP), mesenchymal stem cell (MSC)-derived secretomes, and red-light therapy (RLT) at 633 nm enhance fibroblast activity, collagen synthesis, and angiogenesis, while modulating inflammatory pathways. Dr. Treacy's 2021 modification to include Purosomes from DermaAroma, Italy—derived from bovine colostrum and rich in immunoglobulins, IGF-1, TGF-β, and anti-inflammatory cytokines—further amplifies these regenerative outcomes, promoting tissue repair and countering SASP-driven inflammaging.

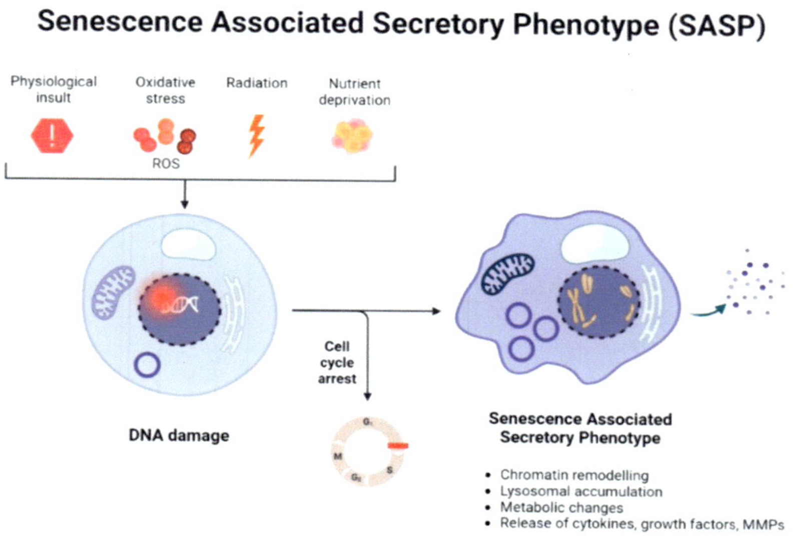

Purosomes from DermaAroma, Italy, derived from bovine colostrum and rich in immunoglobulins, growth factors such as IGF-1 and TGF-β, and anti-inflammatory cytokines, enhance regenerative interventions by delivering bioactive molecules that restore tissue vitality and mitigate inflammaging. These therapies support mesenchymal-to-epithelial transition (MET), minimise excessive epithelial–mesenchymal transition (EMT)-driven fibrosis, and foster an epithelial-friendly microenvironment, aided by RLT through upregulation of antioxidant enzymes and modulation of NF-κB activity.

Therapeutic strategies to balance SASP's dual effects include **senolytics**, which selectively eliminate senescent cells to reduce SASP burden, and **senomorphics**, which modulate SASP factors—such as pro-inflammatory cytokines—without killing cells, thereby preserving their beneficial roles in acute tissue repair. Immune-based approaches aim to enhance the natural clearance of senescent cells by boosting T cell function, while lifestyle interventions—such as antioxidant-rich diets, regular exercise, and minimizing stressors like UV exposure—help reduce senescence onset and SASP-associated tissue damage.

In aesthetic applications, including skin rejuvenation and hair restoration, MSC-derived secretomes and Purosomes deliver growth factors (e.g., FGF, VEGF, IGF-1) and anti-inflammatory cytokines (e.g., IL-10) to reactivate dormant hair follicles, extend the anagen phase, and improve scalp vascularisation. For skin, these therapies stimulate collagen synthesis, improve extracellular matrix organization, and reinforce barrier function. Treatment protocols typically involve topical or intradermal application of secretome-rich formulations—including Purosomes—after microneedling, followed by RLT sessions, with aftercare encompassing additional RLT treatments and protective measures such as scalp care or wound dressings to optimise outcomes.

Regulatory oversight for secretome-based therapies, including bovine colostrum-derived Purosomes, is evolving to ensure safety, efficacy, and standardisation in isolation and processing methods. As of June 2025, future directions include combining secretomes with biomaterials, gene editing technologies (e.g., CRISPR/Cas9), and senolytics to further enhance regenerative outcomes, positioning regenerative aesthetics as a transformative approach to mitigating age-related tissue decline and promoting healthy ageing.

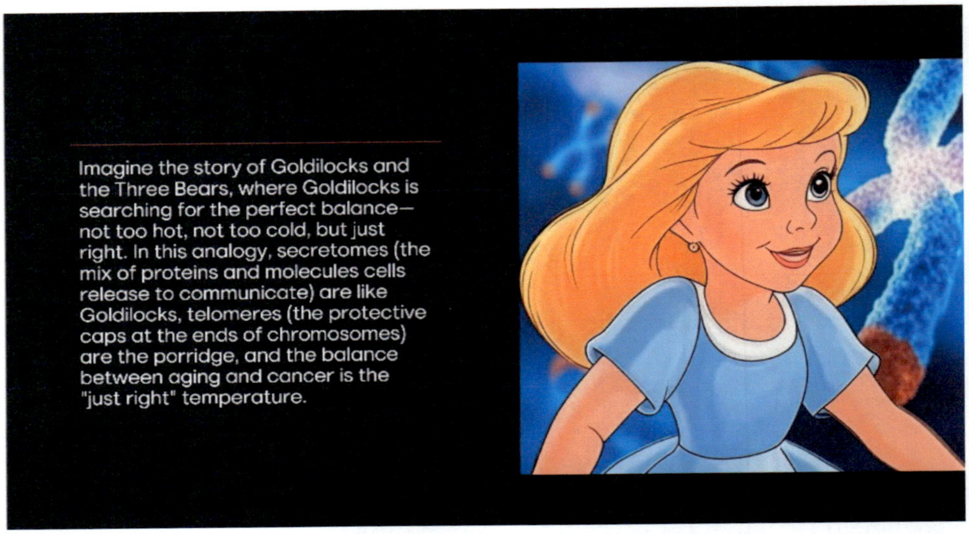

The "Goldilocks phenomenon"

The **"Goldilocks phenomenon,"** a term first coined by Dr. Patrick Treacy, provides a nuanced framework for understanding the balance of telomere dynamics and their influence on ageing and disease, drawing on the familiar fairy tale analogy: conditions must be "just right"—not too hot, not too cold. **Telomeres**, the protective caps at the ends of chromosomes, naturally shorten with each cell division, much like porridge cooling over time. This shortening drives cellular ageing, as cells gradually lose functionality and eventually enter senescence.

Secretomes—complex mixtures of bioactive molecules, including growth factors, cytokines, and exosomes—play a pivotal role in modulating telomere length. They can either support telomere maintenance, akin to keeping the porridge "warm," or allow progressive shortening, letting it "cool." By enhancing telomerase activity, secretomes may prolong cell lifespan, delay age-related decline, and preserve stem cell pluripotency. However, this balance is delicate: excessive telomere elongation—"overheating" the porridge—can promote uncontrolled cell proliferation, a hallmark exploited by cancer cells through telomerase reactivation. Conversely, insufficient maintenance—"cold porridge"—accelerates telomere shortening, limiting cancer risk by curtailing cell survival but hastening ageing and frailty through accelerated tissue degeneration.

Dr. Treacy's 2021 incorporation of **Purosomes** from DermaAroma, Italy—derived from bovine colostrum and rich in growth factors and anti-inflammatory compounds—into his regenerative protocols exemplifies an effort to fine-tune this balance. Purosomes aim to support telomere integrity and cellular health without tipping toward excessive elongation, as of 09:11 PM IST on June 30, 2025.

This framework challenges the oversimplified notion that longer telomeres are universally beneficial. Instead, it underscores the need for precision in secretome-driven interventions, optimising telomere length to mitigate both ageing and cancer risks. In line with the **Goldilocks principle**, the goal is to achieve a state of "just right"—maintaining cellular vitality without promoting uncontrolled proliferation.

Q 31 – Tell me about Cytokines and their role in the body?

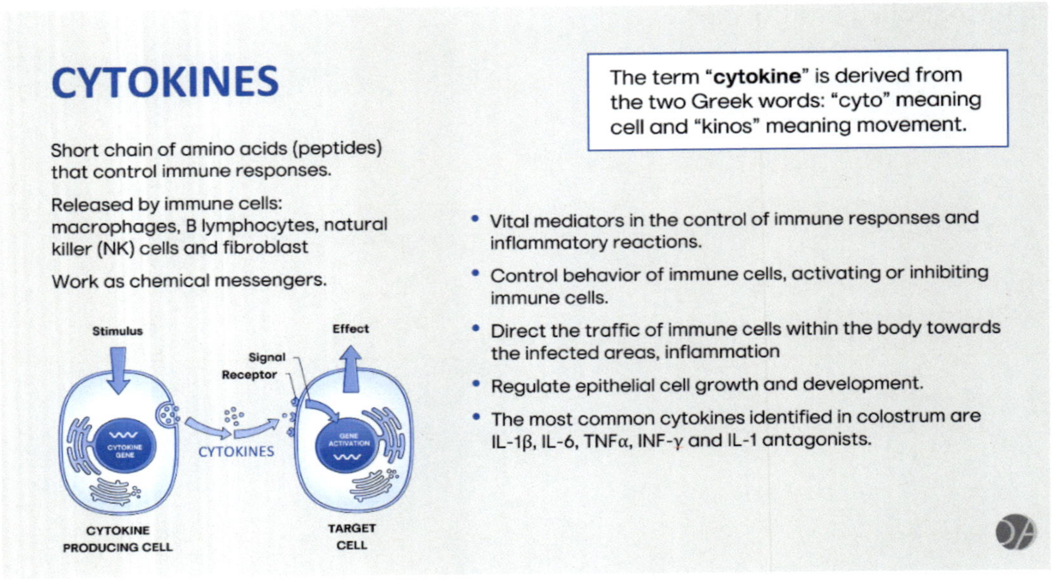

Cytokines are signaling proteins secreted by various cell types—including immune cells such as T cells, macrophages, and dendritic cells—that regulate inflammation, immunity, and tissue homeostasis. Acting as molecular messengers, cytokines bind to specific receptors on target cells to trigger a wide range of biological responses.

Cytokines comprise a diverse family of small proteins and glycoproteins, including **interleukins (ILs), tumor necrosis factors (TNFs), interferons (IFNs), colony-stimulating factors (CSFs), and chemokines**. While primarily secreted by immune cells, non-immune cells such as fibroblasts and endothelial cells can release cytokines in response to injury, infection, or stress. These molecules orchestrate physiological and pathological responses across the body and are central to regenerative and aesthetic medicine. Cytokines exert **autocrine, paracrine, and sometimes endocrine effects**, regulating immune responses through **pro-inflammatory cytokines** (e.g., IL-1, IL-6, TNF-α) that combat infection and **anti-inflammatory cytokines** (e.g., IL-10, TGF-β) that maintain tissue balance. They also influence **cell growth, differentiation, wound healing** through angiogenesis and collagen deposition, antiviral defense via interferons, and chemotaxis guiding immune cell migration.

In ageing tissues, fibroblast senescence and reduced growth factor secretion (e.g., TGF-β, PDGF, FGF) compromise skin integrity and hair follicle health. Cytokines play a dual role in this context: chronic **SASP-driven inflammation** accelerates tissue thinning, wrinkling, and hair loss, whereas regenerative strategies aim to counteract these effects, as of June 30, 2025.

Cytokine classification highlights their versatility:

- **Interleukins** regulate T- and B-cell proliferation and inflammatory responses.

- **TNFs** induce apoptosis in tumor cells and mediate inflammation.
- **Interferons** (e.g., IFN-α, IFN-β for antiviral defense; IFN-γ for adaptive immunity) enhance immune function.
- **CSFs** stimulate hematopoiesis.
- **Chemokines** guide immune cell migration and tissue repair.

Dysregulation of cytokines can have serious consequences. Excessive pro-inflammatory cytokine release can trigger **chronic inflammation, autoimmune disorders** (e.g., rheumatoid arthritis), or **cytokine storms** in severe infections or during certain immunotherapies. Tumor cells may exploit cytokines to suppress immunity or promote angiogenesis, aiding metastasis. In aesthetic contexts, these imbalances accelerate skin ageing and impair wound healing. Therapeutic interventions targeting these pathways include **anti-TNF monoclonal antibodies**, **IL-6 inhibitors**, **G-CSF** to boost white blood cells post-chemotherapy, and **IL-2** to enhance T-cell proliferation in oncology.

Regenerative strategies leverage cytokines to restore tissue function. MSC-derived secretomes deliver **anti-inflammatory cytokines** to mitigate SASP-driven "inflammaging," while **red-light therapy (RLT) at 633 nm** upregulates antioxidant enzymes such as superoxide dismutase (SOD), reducing oxidative stress from reactive oxygen species (ROS) and fostering an epithelial-friendly microenvironment. In **hair restoration**, cytokines such as **TGF-β and VEGF** from secretomes reactivate dormant follicles and enhance scalp vascularization. In **skin rejuvenation**, they stimulate collagen synthesis, improve ECM organization, and restore barrier function.

Treatment protocols typically involve **topical or intradermal application of secretome-rich mixtures post-microneedling**, followed by RLT, with aftercare including additional RLT sessions and protective measures like scalp care or wound dressings to optimize outcomes. Abnormal cytokine levels also serve as **diagnostic biomarkers**, guiding clinical interventions in conditions such as sepsis.

Regulatory oversight for secretome-based therapies, including those delivering cytokines, is evolving to ensure safety, efficacy, and standardization. As of June 2025, **future directions** include combining secretomes with biomaterials, **gene editing tools** (e.g., CRISPR/Cas9), or **senolytics** to enhance regenerative outcomes. Altogether, cytokines represent a cornerstone in regenerative and aesthetic medicine, central to promoting healthy ageing and addressing both inflammatory and tissue-repair challenges.

Q 32 – Tell me about Eotaxin (also known as CCL11) and IL-4 (Interleukin-4)?

Eotaxin (CCL11) and Interleukin-4 (IL-4) are cytokines central to **Th2-mediated immune responses**, primarily recognized for their roles in allergic inflammation and parasitic infections. Beyond their immune functions, both can influence **fibroblast activity** and **collagen synthesis**, with implications for **wound healing, tissue repair, and pathological fibrosis** in regenerative and aesthetic medicine.

Eotaxin (CCL11) is a chemokine best known for **recruiting eosinophils** to sites of inflammation. By promoting a **Th2-rich microenvironment** through eosinophil infiltration, eotaxin indirectly modulates fibroblast behavior. Eosinophils release additional Th2 cytokines, such as **IL-4 and IL-13**, which can influence collagen deposition. In fibrotic conditions—including pulmonary or dermal fibrosis—**elevated eotaxin levels** are associated with increased eosinophil-driven pro-fibrotic activity. While eotaxin does not directly stimulate collagen production, it **creates a milieu that promotes extracellular matrix (ECM) accumulation** and fibrotic remodeling.

Interleukin-4 (IL-4), a hallmark Th2 cytokine essential for **B-cell class switching** and allergic responses, exerts a more direct effect on fibroblasts. IL-4 binds to the **IL-4 receptor** on fibroblasts and myofibroblasts, activating the **STAT6 signaling pathway**, which **upregulates collagen synthesis** and contributes to excessive ECM deposition. This mechanism is implicated in fibrotic diseases affecting the **liver, lungs, and skin**, where dysregulated IL-4 activity drives pathological tissue remodeling.

In regenerative and aesthetic medicine, understanding the **interplay between eotaxin, IL-4, and fibroblast activity** is crucial for balancing **collagen production** and **ECM organization**, optimizing tissue repair while minimizing the risk of fibrosis. As of **June 30, 2025**, insights into these cytokine pathways inform strategies for modulating fibroblast function in therapeutic contexts.

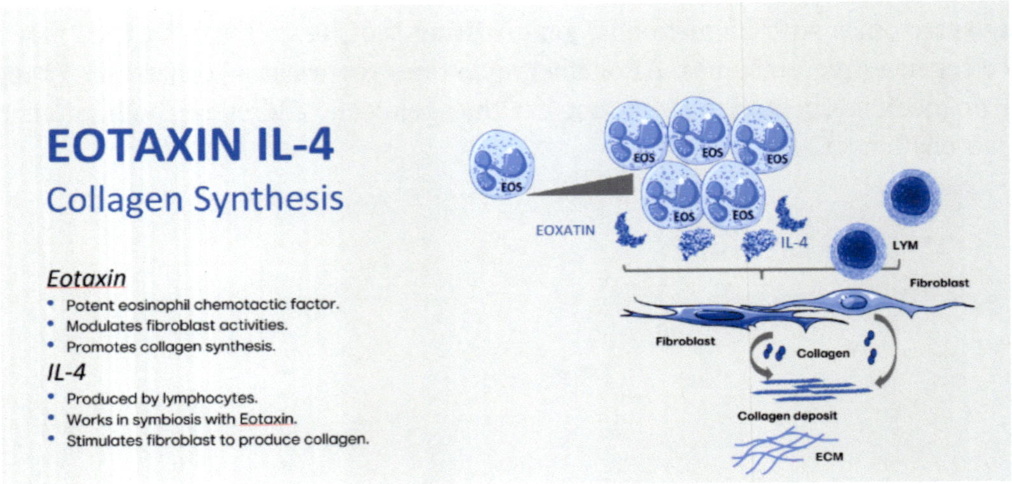

The **synergistic interplay between Eotaxin and IL-4** amplifies their effects, particularly in **chronic inflammatory or allergic conditions** such as atopic dermatitis, asthma, and scleroderma-like fibroses. In these contexts, **Eotaxin-recruited eosinophils** secrete IL-4 and additional growth factors, promoting **fibroblast proliferation and collagen overproduction** within a Th2-dominated environment. While controlled collagen synthesis is beneficial for **wound healing and aesthetic treatments**, chronic Th2 activation can lead to **unwanted fibrosis or scarring**, disrupting tissue architecture. In **hair restoration**, this Th2 bias may impair follicle health by driving inflammation, and in **skin rejuvenation**, it risks compromising barrier function and tissue integrity.

Regenerative strategies mitigate these effects by modulating inflammation and supporting **extracellular matrix (ECM) balance**. Interventions such as **Platelet-Rich Plasma (PRP), mesenchymal stem cell (MSC)-derived secretomes, and red-light therapy (RLT) at 633 nm** act synergistically: secretomes deliver **anti-inflammatory cytokines like IL-10** to counter Th2-driven fibrosis, while RLT enhances antioxidant defenses by upregulating enzymes such as **superoxide dismutase (SOD)**, reducing oxidative stress from **reactive oxygen species (ROS)**.

Targeted therapeutic approaches directly modulate these cytokines to manage fibrotic progression. Anti-IL-4 therapies, including **IL-4 receptor alpha antagonists**, are employed in atopic dermatitis, while **Eotaxin/CCR3 inhibitors** are under investigation for eosinophil-driven inflammation in asthma or sclerotic disorders. In aesthetic applications, these strategies aim to harness **IL-4's collagen-stimulating potential** for controlled tissue repair while preventing excessive fibrosis—a delicate balance essential for maintaining skin and hair health.

Treatment protocols often involve **topical or intradermal application of secretome-rich mixtures post-microneedling**, followed by **RLT**, with aftercare including additional RLT sessions and protective measures such as wound dressings or scalp care to optimise outcomes. **Abnormal levels of Eotaxin and IL-4** can serve as diagnostic biomarkers, guiding clinical decisions. Regulatory oversight for cytokine-modulating therapies is evolving to ensure **safety and efficacy**, with ongoing standardisation addressing variability.

As of **June 2025**, emerging approaches combining **secretomes with biomaterials or gene editing technologies (e.g., CRISPR/Cas9)** show promise for enhancing regenerative outcomes, positioning **cytokine-targeted strategies** as a transformative tool to address **inflammation, fibrosis, and ageing** in both aesthetic and clinical contexts.

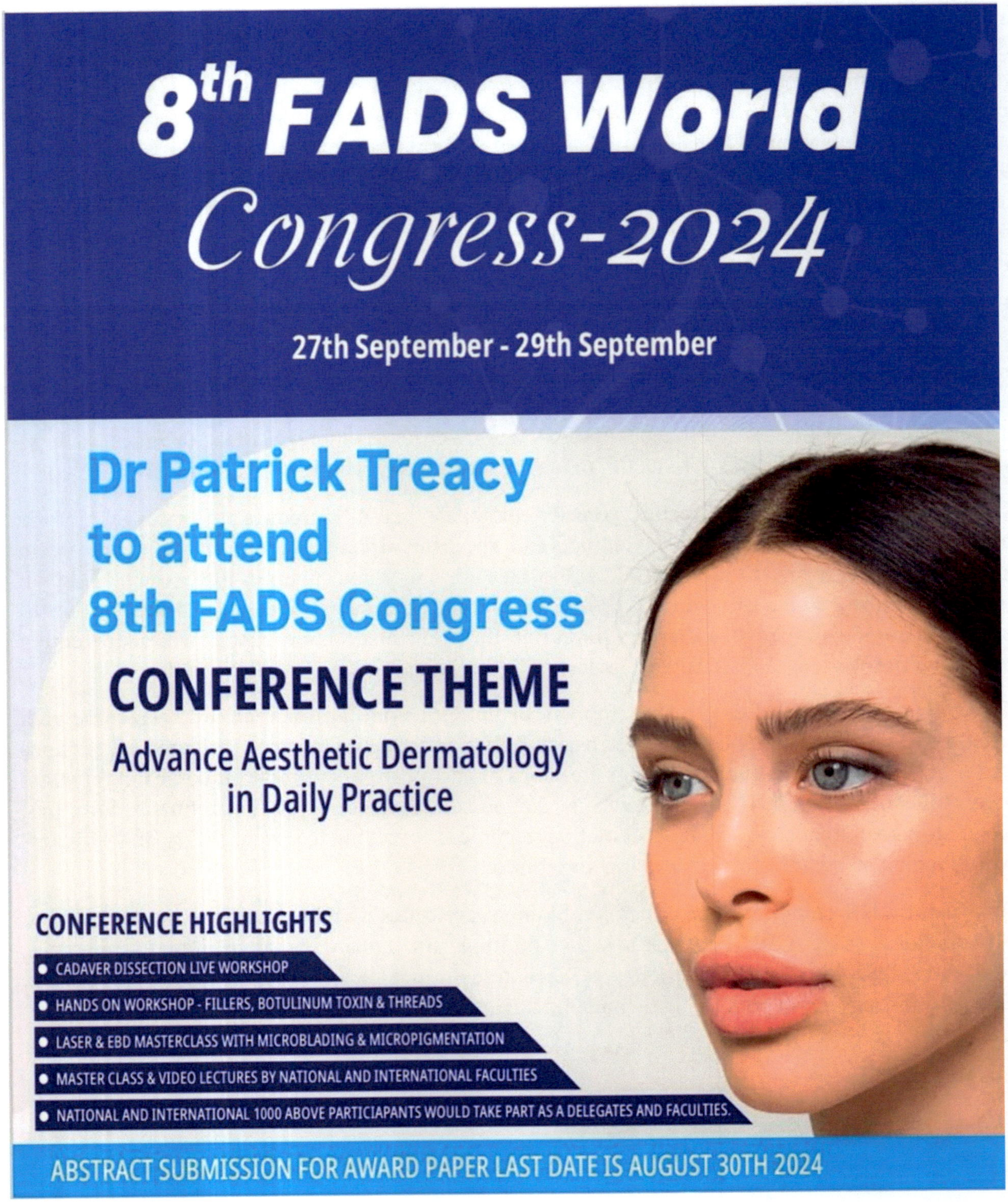

8th FADS World
Congress-2024
27th September - 29th September
Dr Patrick Treacy
to attend
8th FADS Congress
CONFERENCE THEME
Advance Aesthetic Dermatology
in Daily Practice
CONFERENCE HIGHLIGHTS
CADAVER DISSECTION LIVE WORKSHOP
HANDS ON WORKSHOP - FILLERS, BOTULINUM TOXIN & THREADS
LASER & EBD MASTERCLASS WITH MICROBLADING & MICROPIGMENTATION
MASTER CLASS & VIDEO LECTURES BY NATIONAL AND INTERNATIONAL FACULTIES
NATIONAL AND INTERNATIONAL 1000 ABOVE PARTICIAPANTS WOULD TAKE PART AS A DELEGATES AND FACULTIES.
ABSTRACT SUBMISSION FOR AWARD PAPER LAST DATE IS AUGUST 30TH 2024

Q 33 – What are Polynucleotides and how do they work in Aesthetic Medicine?

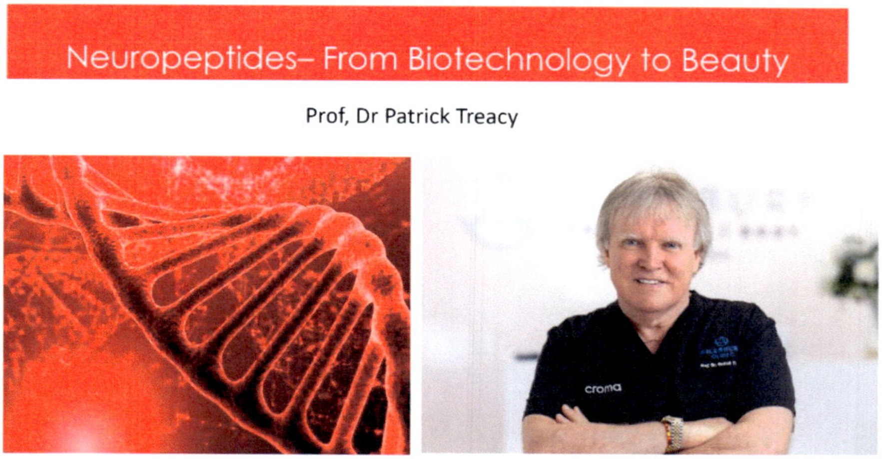

Polynucleotides are long chains of nucleotides—the fundamental building blocks of DNA and RNA. In aesthetic medicine, they typically refer to **fragmented DNA or RNA extracts**, commonly known as **PDRN (Polydeoxyribonucleotide)**, derived from sources such as salmon milt or other biological materials. These fragments have gained attention for their potential to **promote skin regeneration, wound healing, and tissue repair**.

Polynucleotides are **purified DNA or RNA fragments**, processed to remove immunogenic proteins, ensuring safety and compatibility for clinical use. In regenerative aesthetics, they **stimulate fibroblasts**, the cells responsible for producing **collagen and elastin**, thereby enhancing the **extracellular matrix (ECM)**. This activity improves **skin elasticity, hydration, and firmness**, making polynucleotides highly effective for rejuvenation treatments.

These molecules also **upregulate key growth factors** such as **Vascular Endothelial Growth Factor (VEGF)** and **Transforming Growth Factor Beta (TGF-β)**, promoting **angiogenesis and tissue remodelling**. Through the **nucleotide salvage pathway**, polynucleotides provide the raw materials necessary for DNA synthesis, accelerating cellular repair. This mechanism is particularly effective in **wound healing**, where they help **reduce scarring and expedite recovery**, as well as in **post-procedure applications**—for example, after laser treatments or microneedling—by enhancing tissue regeneration.

Polynucleotides also influence **intercellular communication** by modulating growth factor activity. By upregulating VEGF and TGF-β, they enhance **fibroblast signalling**, supporting ECM remodelling and coordinated tissue repair. Their **anti-inflammatory properties** further contribute by reducing local inflammation, creating an environment conducive to healing. This is especially beneficial in **post-procedure recovery** or in tissues under **inflammatory stress**, where polynucleotides help balance immune responses, including the downregulation of pro-inflammatory cytokines.

In aesthetic practice, polynucleotides are typically administered as **"skin boosters" via mesotherapy**, targeting **mild to moderate skin laxity, fine lines, and hydration deficits**, providing **visible improvements with minimal downtime**. They also **accelerate wound closure and reduce scarring**, particularly in chronic wounds or post-surgical contexts. Increasingly, clinicians **combine polynucleotides with modalities** such as **Platelet-Rich Plasma (PRP)** or **microneedling** to enhance collagen stimulation and optimise outcomes.

Polynucleotide injections are also being **explored for scalp health and hair follicle function** in hair restoration, though further research is needed to fully evaluate their efficacy.

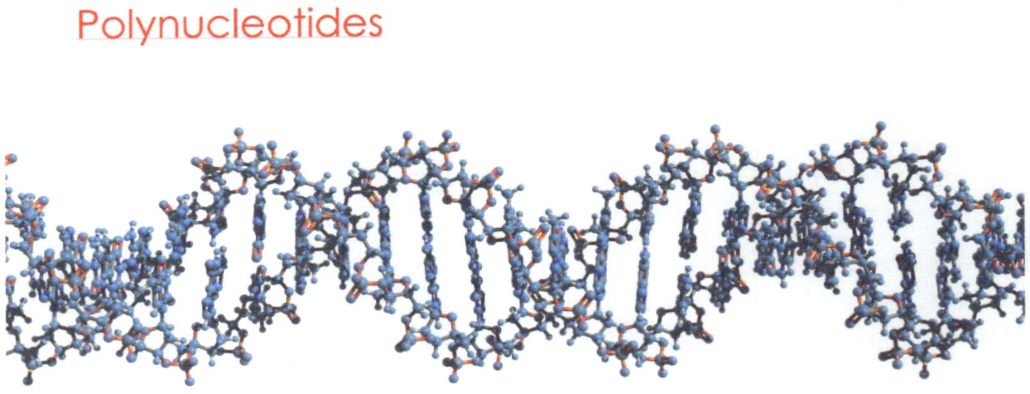

Treatment protocols for polynucleotides vary depending on the specific product and clinical indication. Typically, **multiple sessions spaced two to four weeks apart** are recommended to achieve optimal results. **Ideal candidates** are individuals with **mild to moderate skin laxity, fine lines, or post-procedure healing needs**. Patients with more advanced ageing concerns may require **additional interventions**, such as **dermal fillers or surgical procedures**, to achieve the desired outcomes.

Side effects are generally mild and transient, including **swelling, bruising, or redness at injection sites**, which usually resolve quickly without intervention. **Regulatory oversight** classifies polynucleotide products as **medical devices, cosmetics, or biologics**, depending on local frameworks. Rigorous requirements for **sterility, purity, and traceability**, particularly for **fish-derived formulations**, are in place to ensure patient safety.

Polynucleotides are poised to make **significant advancements in regenerative aesthetics**. A growing body of **clinical trials and case studies** is clarifying **best practices, optimal dosing schedules, and combination strategies**. Research into **hybrid formulations**, such as polynucleotides combined with **peptides or growth factors**, aims to **enhance therapeutic efficacy**.

Advances in **molecular diagnostics and biomarker profiling** hold promise for **personalised treatment regimens**, allowing practitioners to tailor interventions to an individual's **regenerative**

needs and maximise clinical outcomes. While challenges remain in **standardising production and fully validating clinical efficacy**, the **versatility, safety, and regenerative potential** of polynucleotides position them as a **cornerstone of innovative aesthetic medicine**.

Comparison of Secretomes and Polynucleotides

Secretomes, primarily derived from **mesenchymal stem cell (MSC) cultures**, including **adipose tissue** or **umbilical cord** sources, facilitate tissue repair through a **multifaceted regenerative mechanism**. These secretions contain key bioactive molecules such as **vascular endothelial growth factor (VEGF), basic fibroblast growth factor (bFGF), and interleukins**, which collectively **stimulate cell proliferation, migration, and angiogenesis**.

The **extracellular vesicles (EVs)** within secretomes, notably **exosomes**, transfer **microRNAs, proteins, and signaling molecules** to recipient cells, modulating their behavior to **promote tissue regeneration**. In **aesthetic medicine**, secretomes enhance **skin rejuvenation** by **stimulating collagen synthesis, improving elasticity, and reducing pigmentation**, as supported by multiple **cosmeceutical studies**.

Their **immunomodulatory properties** further **attenuate local inflammation**, creating an optimal environment for **healing and tissue repair**, as demonstrated in **preclinical models of wound repair and liver injury**. Unlike cell-based therapies, secretomes offer a **cell-free alternative**, minimizing **risks of immune rejection or tumorigenesis**, while their **standardizable composition** enhances suitability for **clinical applications**.

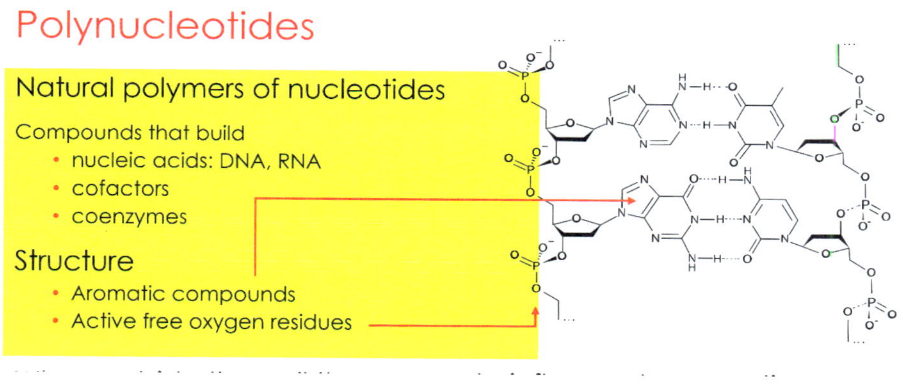

Polynucleotides, in contrast, are more defined in composition, consisting of purified DNA or RNA fragments. Typically **sourced from fish gonads**, these fragments undergo rigorous purification to remove **immunogenic proteins**, ensuring **biocompatibility**. In **aesthetic medicine**, polynucleotides stimulate **fibroblasts**, the cells responsible for **collagen and elastin production**, thereby enhancing the **extracellular matrix (ECM)**. They also **upregulate growth factors** such as **vascular endothelial growth factor (VEGF)** and **transforming growth factor beta (TGF-β)**, promoting **angiogenesis** and **tissue remodelling**.

Through the **nucleotide salvage pathway**, cells can repurpose polynucleotide-derived nucleotides for **DNA synthesis**, accelerating **cellular repair processes**. This mechanism is particularly effective in **skin rejuvenation**, where **injectable polynucleotides**, delivered via **mesotherapy**, improve **hydration, firmness, and elasticity**, and in **wound healing**, where they **reduce scarring** and **expedite tissue recovery**.

The **synergy between secretomes and polynucleotides** lies in their **complementary regenerative actions**. Secretomes provide a **broad spectrum of signalling molecules and extracellular vesicles (EVs)** to orchestrate complex tissue repair, while polynucleotides supply **raw materials for DNA synthesis** and amplify **growth factor activity**. In **skin rejuvenation**, combining **polynucleotide injections with MSC-derived secretomes** may enhance **collagen synthesis, angiogenesis, and ECM remodelling**, yielding superior clinical outcomes. Similarly, in **wound healing**, the **immunomodulatory effects of secretomes** complement the **tissue-closure and repair properties of polynucleotides**, as demonstrated in **preclinical models of excisional wounds**.

Emerging combination therapies, such as pairing these agents with **platelet-rich plasma (PRP)** or **microneedling**, further amplify regenerative potential, offering **tailored solutions** for aesthetic and clinical indications. Treatment protocols are **patient-specific**: polynucleotide regimens typically involve **multiple sessions spaced 2–4 weeks apart**, with **minimal side effects** such as transient swelling or bruising. Secretome applications, often requiring **Good Manufacturing Practice (GMP) production** for consistency, are similarly **well-tolerated** but demand **standardised protocols** to ensure efficacy. Both modalities are ideal for **mild to moderate skin laxity or post-procedure recovery**, though **severe ageing may necessitate adjunctive treatments** such as dermal fillers or laser therapy.

Regulatory oversight ensures product **safety, sterility, and purity**, particularly for **fish-derived polynucleotides and MSC secretomes**. Looking forward, the **integration of secretomes and polynucleotides** holds **transformative potential**. Research into **hybrid formulations**, such as **polynucleotides combined with peptides** or **preconditioned secretomes enriched via hypoxic culture**, aims to **optimise therapeutic outcomes**. **Personalised regimens**, guided by **biomarker profiling**, may further refine treatment efficacy. While challenges remain in **standardisation and clinical validation**, ongoing **clinical trials** continue to clarify their utility, particularly in **novel applications like hair restoration**.

Conclusion

Polynucleotides, especially short DNA/RNA fragments like **PDRN**, have emerged as a **versatile tool in regenerative aesthetics**, promoting **collagen synthesis, tissue repair, and anti-inflammatory effects**. Often sourced from **salmon milt** for its **high DNA content and low immunogenicity**, these agents are applied in **facial rejuvenation, wound healing, and post-procedure recovery**. As research advances and protocols become more **standardised**, polynucleotide-based therapies are poised to play an increasingly **prominent role in regenerative aesthetic medicine**, complementing cell-based and secretome-driven approaches.

Q 34 – Tell me about the antioxidative effects, moisturisation and proliferation effects of PDRNs?

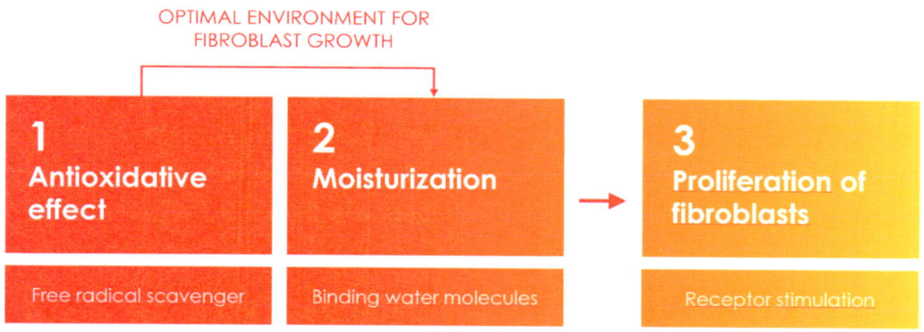

In aesthetic medicine, polynucleotides (PDRNs) excel at mitigating oxidative stress, a key driver of skin ageing. Reactive oxygen species (ROS), generated during normal cellular metabolism, damage proteins, lipids, and DNA, accelerating ageing and impairing tissue repair. PDRNs counteract these effects by modulating cellular pathways and potentially upregulating protective enzymes, reducing ROS-induced damage. Their anti-inflammatory properties further complement this effect by regulating pro-inflammatory cytokines, fostering a balanced cellular environment that indirectly mitigates oxidative stress.

As DNA fragments, PDRNs also supply nucleotide precursors via the salvage pathway, enabling cells to repair DNA damage in rapidly dividing or regenerating tissues, such as during wound healing or post-procedure recovery. Additionally, PDRNs enhance skin hydration by stimulating keratinocytes and fibroblasts, which strengthen epidermal integrity and improve water retention. Activation of fibroblasts further boosts the production of glycosaminoglycans (GAGs), including hyaluronic acid, which are vital for maintaining dermal moisture. When combined with microneedling or platelet-rich plasma (PRP), PDRNs enhance the penetration and retention of hydrating agents in deeper skin layers. This combination contributes to visibly smoother, firmer, and more supple skin, making PDRNs highly effective in rejuvenation therapies.

The regenerative potential of PDRNs is closely tied to their proliferative effects on fibroblasts. By stimulating fibroblast proliferation, PDRNs drive the synthesis of collagen, elastin, and other extracellular matrix (ECM) components, enhancing skin firmness and reducing fine lines. They also upregulate vascular endothelial growth factor (VEGF), promoting angiogenesis to ensure adequate nutrient and oxygen delivery to support active cell proliferation. The nucleotide salvage pathway accelerates tissue renewal by supplying nucleotides for DNA replication in rapidly dividing cells, particularly fibroblasts during wound healing.

PDRNs are therefore essential in skin rejuvenation, scar reduction, and post-procedure recovery, with emerging potential for hair restoration, pending further research. Treatment protocols typically involve multiple sessions spaced two to four weeks apart to achieve cumulative benefits. Ideal candidates include patients with mild to moderate skin laxity, fine lines, or post-procedure healing needs, whereas severe ageing may require adjunctive interventions such as dermal fillers. Side effects are minimal, typically limited to mild swelling or bruising at injection sites, which resolve quickly.

Regulatory frameworks classify polynucleotides as medical devices, cosmetics, or biologics, depending on local regulations, with strict standards for sterility, purity, and traceability, particularly for fish-derived formulations. Polynucleotides are poised to make significant advancements in regenerative aesthetics. Ongoing clinical trials are refining best practices, dosing, and combination strategies, while research into hybrid formulations with peptides or growth factors aims to enhance efficacy. Advances in molecular diagnostics may enable personalised regimens tailored to individual regenerative needs.

Polydeoxyribonucleotides (PDRNs) in Cellular Renewal and Tissue Regeneration

PDRNs play a pivotal role in cellular renewal and tissue regeneration, making them a cornerstone of advanced aesthetic and regenerative therapies. Their capacity to stimulate cellular proliferation and support tissue repair is driven by multiple mechanisms, including fibroblast activation, angiogenesis, and nucleotide salvage pathways. Collectively, these processes enhance tissue vitality, structural integrity, and healing efficiency, offering substantial benefits for skin rejuvenation and wound repair.

Fibroblast Stimulation and Collagen Synthesis

A defining feature of PDRN therapy is its ability to promote fibroblast proliferation, a critical process for maintaining and repairing the extracellular matrix (ECM). Fibroblasts are the primary cells responsible for synthesizing collagen, elastin, and other ECM proteins, which provide structural support and elasticity to the skin and connective tissues. PDRNs act by binding to purinergic receptors (e.g., A2A adenosine receptors), triggering intracellular signaling cascades that enhance fibroblast activity and proliferation.

This increased fibroblast activity results in a marked upregulation of collagen types I and III, which are essential for skin firmness and resilience. Enhanced elastin synthesis contributes to improved elasticity, reducing the appearance of fine lines, wrinkles, and sagging. Clinical studies, such as those published in Dermatologic Therapy (2024), demonstrate that PDRN injections improve skin texture and firmness in patients with photoaged skin, with effects lasting up to six months post-treatment.

The boost in ECM production also accelerates wound healing, making PDRNs valuable for treating chronic wounds, scars, and post-surgical tissue recovery. For example, a 2023 study in the Journal of Tissue Engineering showed that PDRN therapy reduced healing time in diabetic ulcers by 20–30% compared to standard care. Beyond aesthetics, fibroblast stimulation by PDRNs supports broader regenerative applications, such as tendon repair and cartilage regeneration, where

ECM integrity is critical. This versatility positions PDRNs as a transformative agent in both cosmetic and medical contexts.

Angiogenesis

Polydeoxyribonucleotides (PDRNs) significantly enhance **angiogenesis**, the formation of new blood vessels, which is essential for delivering **oxygen, nutrients, and immune cells** to regenerating tissues. By upregulating **vascular endothelial growth factor (VEGF)** expression, PDRNs stimulate **endothelial cell proliferation and migration**, promoting robust **capillary formation**. This ensures a consistent blood supply to support metabolically active cells during **tissue repair and regeneration**.

Enhanced **microcirculation** accelerates wound healing and sustains long-term tissue health. In aesthetic applications, improved blood flow contributes to a **radiant complexion** and supports nutrient delivery to the **dermis**, enhancing overall skin vitality. Research published in *Aesthetic Plastic Surgery* (2024) demonstrated that PDRN-treated skin exhibited a **15–20% increase in microvascular density** compared to controls, correlating with improved skin tone and reduced signs of aging. In **regenerative medicine**, PDRN-induced angiogenesis is critical for **burn recovery** and **chronic wound management**, where adequate vascularization prevents tissue necrosis and promotes faster recovery.

Moreover, PDRNs' angiogenic effects **synergize with other growth factors**, such as those found in **platelet-rich plasma (PRP)**, amplifying regenerative potential. This synergy is particularly beneficial in **combination therapies**, where PDRNs and PRP are applied together to enhance tissue repair in procedures like **hair restoration** or **scar revision**.

Nucleotide Salvage Pathway Support

Rapidly dividing cells, such as **fibroblasts** and **keratinocytes** during tissue repair, require a steady supply of nucleotides for **DNA replication** and **RNA synthesis**. PDRNs, derived from **salmon sperm DNA**, provide a rich source of **deoxyribonucleotides** that cells can repurpose via the **nucleotide salvage pathway**. This pathway bypasses the energy-intensive **de novo nucleotide synthesis**, accelerating **cell division and tissue regeneration**.

By supplying nucleotide precursors, PDRNs reduce the **metabolic burden** on cells, enabling faster proliferation and repair. This mechanism is particularly effective in tissues with **high cell turnover**, such as the **epidermis**, or during wound healing when nucleotide demand increases. A 2023 study in *Regenerative Medicine* reported that PDRN supplementation **increased fibroblast proliferation by up to 25% in vitro**, attributed to enhanced nucleotide availability. In vivo, this translates to **faster epithelialization** and **reduced scar formation** in cutaneous wounds.

Additionally, the salvage pathway supports **DNA repair** in stressed or damaged cells, protecting against **mutations induced by oxidative stress or UV exposure**. This dual role in **cell proliferation and repair** makes PDRNs a powerful tool for both **aesthetic rejuvenation** and **therapeutic tissue regeneration**, with applications ranging from **skin revitalization** to **musculoskeletal repair**.

Synergistic Effects with the Cellular Microenvironment

PDRNs modulate the **cellular microenvironment** to optimize regenerative outcomes. By enhancing the expression of **growth factors** such as **transforming growth factor-beta (TGF-β)** and **insulin-like growth factor-1 (IGF-1)**, PDRNs create a **pro-regenerative milieu** that supports sustained cellular activity. These growth factors further amplify **fibroblast** and **keratinocyte function**, reinforcing **ECM production** and tissue remodeling.

PDRNs also influence **immune cell behavior**, promoting a shift from **pro-inflammatory (M1) to anti-inflammatory (M2) macrophage phenotypes**. This immunomodulatory effect reduces chronic inflammation in damaged tissues, creating an environment more conducive to regeneration. In aesthetic applications, this translates to **reduced post-treatment swelling** and **faster recovery**, as noted in clinical trials combining PDRNs with **microneedling** (*Journal of Cosmetic Dermatology*, 2024). In regenerative medicine, immunomodulation is critical for conditions such as **osteoarthritis**, where PDRNs have shown promise in **reducing joint inflammation** and promoting **cartilage repair**.

Conclusion

Polydeoxyribonucleotides (PDRNs) represent a **transformative advancement** in **aesthetic and regenerative medicine**, offering a **multifaceted approach** to tissue repair and rejuvenation that extends beyond traditional wound healing. Their **antioxidative properties** mitigate cellular damage by reducing **reactive oxygen species (ROS)** and modulating **inflammatory pathways**, creating a protective environment for healthy tissue function.

Simultaneously, PDRNs enhance **skin hydration** by strengthening the **epidermal barrier** and boosting **glycosaminoglycan (GAG)** production, particularly **hyaluronic acid**, which is essential for maintaining **moisture and skin plumpness**. When combined with treatments such as **microneedling, PRP, or LED phototherapy**, PDRNs improve **absorption and extend results**, providing superior moisturization.

The **proliferative effects** of PDRNs—driven by **fibroblast stimulation, angiogenesis, and nucleotide salvage pathway support**—underpin their ability to **rejuvenate skin and soft tissues**. By promoting **collagen and elastin synthesis**, PDRNs restore skin firmness, reduce visible signs of aging, and accelerate wound healing across both **cosmetic** and **medical** applications. Their angiogenic properties ensure **optimal nutrient delivery** to regenerating tissues, while nucleotide availability supports **rapid cellular turnover and DNA repair**.

Furthermore, PDRNs' ability to **modulate the cellular microenvironment and immune response** enhances their regenerative potential, making them a versatile tool for conditions ranging from **photoaged skin** to **chronic wounds** and **musculoskeletal injuries**. In clinical practice, PDRNs are increasingly integrated into **multimodal treatment protocols**, leveraging their synergy with technologies like **PRP, laser therapy, and photobiomodulation** to achieve superior outcomes. Studies as of **June 2025** indicate that PDRN-based therapies can **reduce recovery time by 15–25%** compared to standalone treatments, while improving **skin texture, elasticity**, and **patient satisfaction**.

In **regenerative medicine**, PDRNs play roles in **cartilage repair, tendon regeneration, and burn recovery**, highlighting their broader therapeutic potential. While specific techniques like the **PLUS Technique** are not explicitly linked to PDRNs in available literature, the principles of combining **biological agents** with **phototherapeutic interventions** reflect current innovations in the field, exemplified by practitioners such as **Dr. Patrick Treacy**. Whether used **alone or in combination**, PDRNs provide a scientifically grounded, clinically validated approach to **enhancing tissue regeneration**, **improving aesthetic outcomes**, and **promoting overall tissue health**, positioning them as a **cornerstone of modern regenerative medicine**.

Q 35 – Tell me more about the PDRN Anti-Oxidative Effect on Free Radicals?

Free radicals, commonly referred to as **reactive oxygen species (ROS)**, are natural byproducts of **cellular metabolism**, particularly within the **mitochondria**, where oxygen is utilized for **ATP production**. Although cells are equipped with **intrinsic defense mechanisms**—including antioxidant enzymes, **glutathione**, and **catalase**—excessive ROS can overwhelm these protective systems, resulting in **oxidative stress**.

Chronic oxidative stress triggers a cascade of cellular damage: it promotes **lipid peroxidation**, compromising **cell membrane integrity**; **denatures proteins**, impairing enzymatic and structural functions; and induces **DNA damage**, increasing the risk of mutations and impaired cellular replication. Collectively, these effects **accelerate skin aging**, hinder **tissue repair**, and contribute to a range of **degenerative processes** across multiple organ systems.

1 Antioxidative Effect

Free radical scavenger

Modulation of Key Antioxidant Pathways: One of the body's primary defenses against oxidative stress is mediated by **Nuclear factor erythroid 2–related factor 2 (Nrf2)**. Upon activation, Nrf2 translocates to the nucleus and binds to the **Antioxidant Response Element (ARE)**, triggering the transcription of genes encoding critical **antioxidant enzymes**, including **heme oxygenase-1 (HO-1)** and **glutathione S-transferase**.

Polydeoxyribonucleotides (PDRNs) may enhance or stabilize Nrf2 activity through several mechanisms: by **reducing inhibitory inflammatory mediators**, by **creating a cellular environment conducive to Nrf2 activation**, or by supporting signaling pathways that maintain Nrf2 nuclear translocation. The result is **upregulated expression of antioxidant enzymes** and more efficient **neutralization of reactive oxygen species (ROS)**.

Conversely, **NF-κB (nuclear factor kappa B)** is a transcription factor that promotes the expression of numerous **pro-inflammatory and pro-oxidant genes** under stress conditions. By **modulating NF-κB activity**—either indirectly via balancing anti-inflammatory cytokines or directly inhibiting its signaling—PDRNs can **attenuate the production of ROS** and reduce oxidative damage, complementing Nrf2-mediated antioxidant defense.

Aromatic compounds serve as **free radical scavengers**.
The enzyme-related degradation of polynucleotide molecules can lead to an amplification of protective activities against **free radicals**.

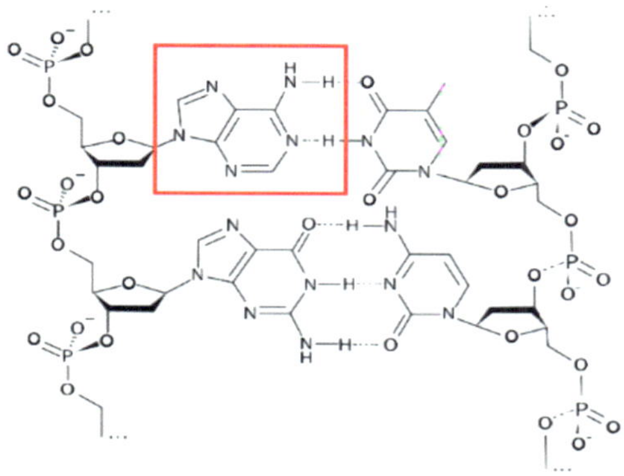

Upregulation of Protective Enzymes: Cells depend on enzymes such as **superoxide dismutase (SOD)**, **catalase**, and **glutathione peroxidase** to neutralize reactive oxygen species (ROS) and prevent oxidative damage. Early **in vitro** and **in vivo** studies suggest that **polydeoxyribonucleotide (PDRN)** treatment can enhance the **activity and expression** of these enzymes. This effect is likely mediated by **stabilized gene transcription under reduced inflammatory conditions** and a more favorable **extracellular microenvironment**. PDRNs may also indirectly sustain intracellular **glutathione (GSH) levels**, the primary cellular antioxidant, by **supporting cellular energy balance** and reducing the metabolic drain caused by chronic inflammation. The resulting improvement in antioxidant capacity lowers ROS burden, mitigating oxidative damage to **cell membranes, proteins, and DNA**.

Improved Cellular Repair and DNA Salvage: PDRNs provide short-chain nucleotides that cells can reutilize through the **nucleotide salvage pathway**. Under oxidative stress, the incidence of **DNA damage increases**, and readily available nucleotides facilitate more efficient repair via mechanisms such as **base excision repair**. Accelerated repair of oxidative lesions helps **prevent the accumulation of mutations** and preserves cellular function. When DNA damage becomes excessive, cells may trigger **programmed cell death (apoptosis)**; by enabling timely repair, PDRNs can **prevent unnecessary cell loss**, maintaining tissue integrity and supporting regenerative processes.

Neutralizing Free Radicals:
Polynucleotides, as fragments of DNA or RNA, contain bases that can react with reactive oxygen species (ROS) and neutralize them. By donating electrons, they stabilise these free radicals and prevent them from causing cellular damage.

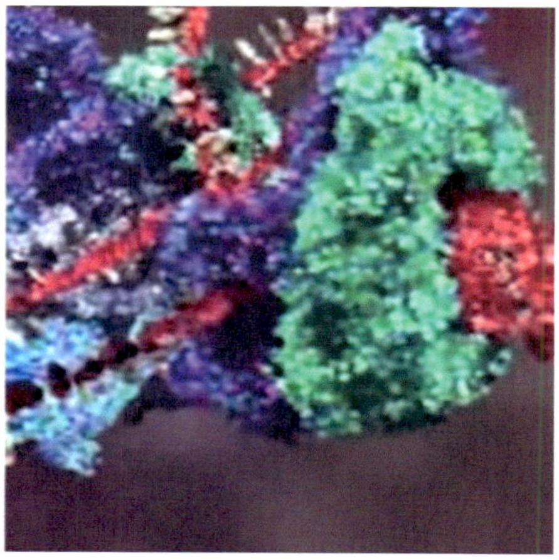

Anti-Inflammatory and Immunomodulatory Effects

Cytokine Balance:

Oxidative stress is often intensified by a **pro-inflammatory environment**, characterized by elevated cytokines such as **TNF-α** and **IL-6**. Studies indicate that **polydeoxyribonucleotides (PDRNs)** can **reduce pro-inflammatory mediators** while **enhancing anti-inflammatory signals**, thereby restoring a more balanced immune response. Inflammatory cells, including **neutrophils and macrophages**, generate ROS as part of their pathogen-killing activity; by modulating inflammation, PDRNs help **limit excessive ROS release**, protecting surrounding tissues from collateral damage.

Improved Tissue Perfusion:

Chronic oxidative stress can impair **microcirculation**, reducing oxygen and nutrient delivery to tissues. PDRN-induced **angiogenesis**, often mediated via **VEGF upregulation**, enhances blood flow, supporting nutrient and oxygen supply, removing metabolic byproducts, and sustaining antioxidant defenses. This optimized microenvironment promotes **cellular metabolism** and resilience against oxidative damage.

Reduced Photoaging:

Ultraviolet (UV) radiation is a major source of ROS in the skin, contributing to **collagen degradation, elastin breakdown, and hyperpigmentation**. By strengthening the skin's **antioxidant capacity**, PDRNs can attenuate UV-induced damage, preserving structural proteins and maintaining dermal integrity.

Accelerated Wound Healing:

Oxidative stress is a key factor in delayed wound closure. By fostering a healthier oxidative balance, PDRNs **enhance re-epithelialization**, reduce scarring, and promote **robust collagen deposition** without triggering excessive inflammation. Their regenerative effects can be further potentiated when combined with adjunctive therapies, such as **microneedling, laser treatments, or exosome-based therapies**, each of which may stimulate complementary antioxidant and repair pathways.

Multifaceted Regenerative Mechanisms:

PDRNs offer more than a substrate for collagen synthesis—they provide a **protective antioxidative and immunomodulatory dimension**. By modulating key transcription factors such as **Nrf2** and **NF-κB**, upregulating antioxidant enzymes, supporting nucleotide salvage pathways, and reducing chronic inflammation, PDRNs establish an environment in which cells are better equipped to **neutralize ROS**. The overall effect is **reduced oxidative damage**, improved cellular function, and a **slower progression of skin aging**.

Enhanced Hydration and Skin Function:

In addition to their regenerative and antioxidant properties, PDRNs improve the skin's **intrinsic ability to retain moisture**, supporting glycosaminoglycan and hyaluronic acid production. This results in **enhanced hydration, increased elasticity, and healthier overall skin function**, reinforcing their growing significance in **regenerative and aesthetic medicine**.

Q 36 – How do polynucleotides hydrate the skin?

2 Moisturization

Binding water molecules

Polynucleotides (PDRNs) and Skin Hydration: Mechanisms of Moisture Enhancement

Fibroblast Activation and Glycosaminoglycan Synthesis:

Polynucleotides (PDRNs) stimulate **dermal fibroblasts**, promoting the production of **glycosaminoglycans (GAGs)**, including **hyaluronic acid (HA)**, as well as other extracellular matrix (ECM) components. GAGs are highly hydrophilic molecules capable of binding and retaining water, so their increased synthesis directly enhances **skin hydration, elasticity, and suppleness**.

Collagen Support and ECM Integrity:

By supporting fibroblast activity and **collagen synthesis**, PDRNs reinforce the **dermal scaffold**, which contributes to **better water retention** and reduced **trans-epidermal water loss (TEWL)**. Additionally, PDRNs facilitate **keratinocyte turnover and organization**, strengthening the **stratum corneum**, the skin's outermost layer. A healthier epidermal barrier helps **lock in moisture**, maintaining plump, hydrated skin cells.

Anti-Inflammatory Effects:

Chronic inflammation can compromise barrier lipids and structural proteins, increasing water loss and reducing hydration. PDRNs exhibit **anti-inflammatory and immunomodulatory effects**, mitigating these disruptions and supporting a **more intact epidermal barrier**, thereby promoting long-term moisture balance.

Enhanced Microcirculation and Nutrient Delivery:

PDRNs promote **angiogenesis** by upregulating growth factors such as **vascular endothelial growth factor (VEGF)**, improving **microcirculation** within the dermis. Enhanced blood flow ensures **optimal delivery of oxygen and nutrients** to skin cells, supporting the production of hydration-related molecules such as HA and ceramides. Improved microcirculation also facilitates the **removal of metabolic waste**, reducing oxidative stress and inflammation, both of which can impair the skin's ability to retain moisture.

Summary:

Through a combination of **fibroblast stimulation, ECM reinforcement, anti-inflammatory action, and improved microcirculation**, PDRNs enhance **skin hydration, barrier function, and overall dermal health**, making them a powerful tool in regenerative and aesthetic dermatology.

Hydration and Skin Plumping: By attracting water molecules, polynucleotides help maintain optimal skin hydration. This results in plumper, more supple skin, which can also contribute indirectly to a reduction in the appearance of fine lines and wrinkles.

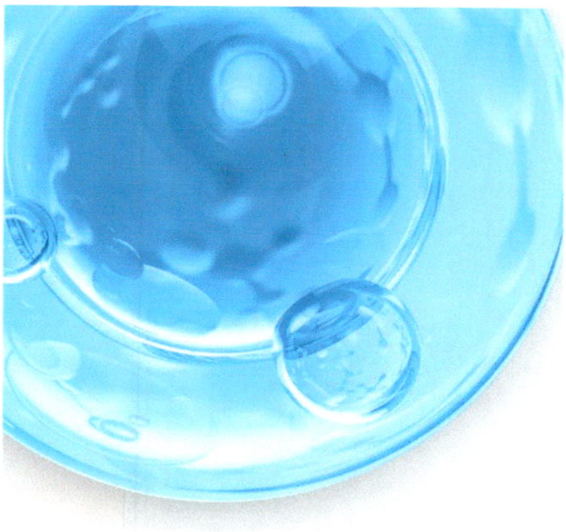

Nucleotide Salvage and Cellular Health:

Polynucleotides (PDRNs), as fragments of DNA or RNA, can be metabolized into nucleotide building blocks. Skin cells can reuse these nucleotides via the **nucleotide salvage pathway** for DNA repair and cell turnover, supporting **healthy, metabolically active cells**. Well-functioning cells are better equipped to produce **structural proteins and glycosaminoglycans (GAGs)**, including hyaluronic acid, which are critical for maintaining **hydration and skin resilience**.

Reduced Cellular Stress:

By facilitating DNA repair and potentially enhancing **antioxidant defenses**, polynucleotides help mitigate **oxidative stress** and delay **cellular senescence**—both of which are associated with decreased production of natural moisturizing factors. Integrating PDRNs with **microneedling** can enhance penetration, while **platelet-rich plasma (PRP)** provides additional growth factors. Together, these interventions synergistically stimulate **collagen and GAG synthesis**, resulting in sustained improvements in skin hydration.

Complementary Regimens:

Polynucleotide-based serums or creams can be combined with **moisturizers, peptides, and ceramide-rich formulations** to create a comprehensive skin care regimen, maximizing hydration and barrier support.

Key Takeaways:

- **Hydration through ECM Support:** PDRNs stimulate fibroblasts to produce **GAGs** (particularly hyaluronic acid) and **collagen**, enhancing the skin's water-retention capacity.
- **Barrier Strengthening:** By supporting epidermal integrity, PDRNs reduce **trans-epidermal water loss (TEWL)** and may mitigate inflammation that can compromise hydration.
- **Optimized Microenvironment:** Enhanced **angiogenesis, cellular repair, and antioxidant support** create favorable conditions for robust, well-hydrated skin.

Q 37 – How Do Polynucleotides stimulate fibroblast proliferation?

3

Proliferation of Fibroblasts

OPTIMAL HYDRATION OF ECM

DNA SALVAGE

A2 Receptor stimulation

Polynucleotides (PDRNs) and Fibroblast Proliferation

Polynucleotides—short fragments of DNA or RNA, commonly referred to as PDRNs—support **fibroblast proliferation** through multiple, interrelated mechanisms:

1. **Nucleotide Supply via the Salvage Pathway:** Once metabolized, polynucleotides provide nucleotides that cells can repurpose through the **nucleotide salvage pathway**. Fibroblasts, which require a continuous supply of nucleotides for **DNA replication**, benefit from this readily available pool, enabling more efficient entry into the cell cycle and sustained mitotic activity.

2. **Stimulation of Growth Factor Release:** Polynucleotides may trigger fibroblasts and surrounding cells to release **growth factors** such as **FGF (fibroblast growth factor)** and **PDGF (platelet-derived growth factor)**, as well as signaling cytokines. These molecules act in an autocrine and paracrine manner, further enhancing fibroblast proliferation and activity.

3. **Improvement of the Cellular Microenvironment:** By reducing **inflammation** and supporting tissue repair, polynucleotides create a more favorable environment for fibroblasts. This immunomodulatory effect helps fibroblasts respond more effectively to proliferation cues and external signals.

4. **Angiogenesis and Nutrient Support:** Polynucleotides upregulate **VEGF (vascular endothelial growth factor)**, promoting angiogenesis and improved microcirculation. Enhanced blood flow delivers **oxygen and nutrients** to fibroblasts, which is critical for sustaining growth, energy production, and progression through the cell cycle.

5. **Inflammation Modulation:** Chronic or excessive inflammation can impair fibroblast function. Polynucleotides help balance inflammatory mediators, thereby protecting fibroblasts from the detrimental effects of oxidative stress and inflammatory signaling.

Collectively, these mechanisms enable polynucleotides to **prime fibroblasts for optimal proliferation and ECM production**, supporting tissue regeneration, wound healing, and skin rejuvenation.

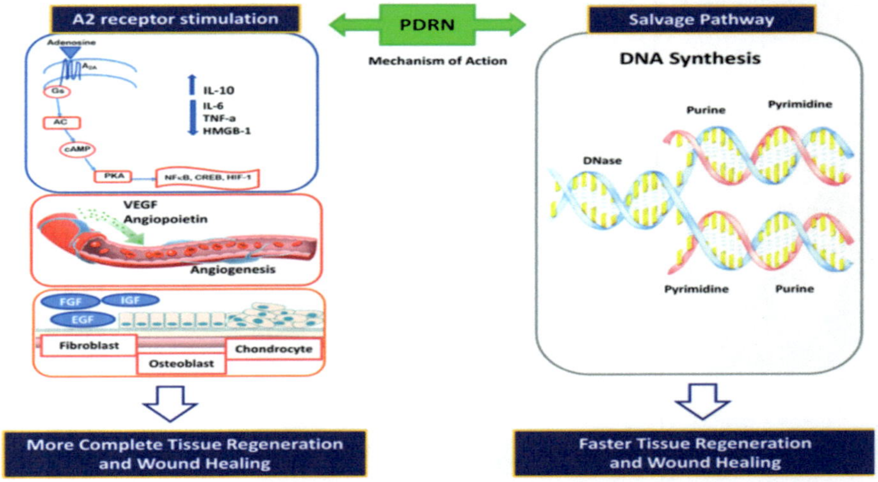

DNA Repair Enhancement and Fibroblast Activation

Polynucleotides can facilitate the repair of damaged DNA in fibroblasts, supporting genomic integrity and reducing the likelihood that cells will pause or exit the cell cycle due to DNA damage. By enhancing DNA repair mechanisms, polynucleotides help maintain a **proliferative fibroblast population**, critical for tissue regeneration and skin rejuvenation.

Some studies indicate that polynucleotides may also reduce **reactive oxygen species (ROS)** levels or upregulate cellular antioxidant defenses, thereby minimizing oxidative damage and further supporting fibroblast survival and function. Additionally, nucleic acid fragments or their metabolites may interact with **purinergic receptors (e.g., A2A)** or **toll-like receptors (TLRs)** on the cell surface. Activation of these receptors can trigger **MAPK/ERK signaling pathways**, leading to increased expression of genes involved in the fibroblast cell cycle, proliferation, and extracellular matrix (ECM) synthesis.

Overall, polynucleotides promote fibroblast proliferation and activity through multiple complementary mechanisms: supporting DNA synthesis, enhancing growth factor signaling, reducing inflammatory stress, and stimulating tissue repair pathways. The cumulative effect is a **healthier, more active fibroblast population**, capable of producing collagen, elastin, and other ECM components essential for skin firmness, elasticity, and overall tissue integrity.

Q 38 – How do polynucleotides work with A2 skin receptors?

Polydeoxyribonucleotides (PDRNs) have been demonstrated in multiple studies to mediate aspects of their regenerative and pro-healing effects through **activation of adenosine A2 receptors**, particularly the **A2A subtype**, on target cells such as fibroblasts and endothelial cells. The following overview summarizes the mechanisms by which A2A receptor activation contributes to tissue repair and regeneration:

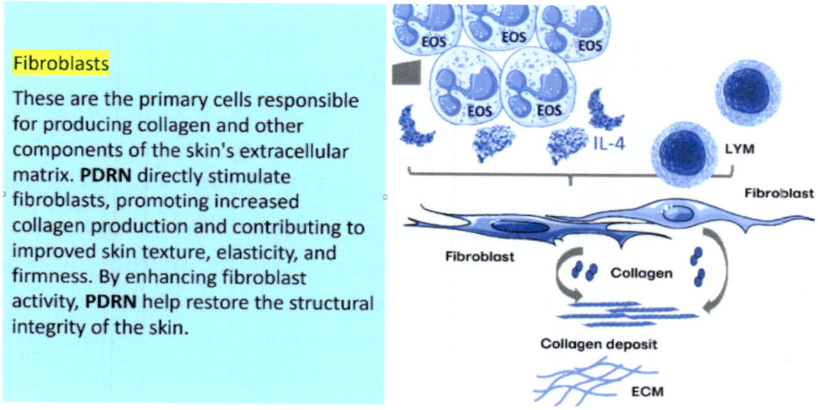

A2 Receptor Family: Adenosine receptors are G protein–coupled receptors (GPCRs) comprising several subtypes, including A1, A2A, A2B, and A3. The A2A and A2B subtypes are particularly implicated in **vasodilation, immune modulation, and tissue regeneration**. A2 receptors, especially A2A, primarily couple to **Gs proteins**, which activate adenylyl cyclase and increase intracellular **cAMP levels**. Elevated cAMP subsequently stimulates **protein kinase A (PKA)** and downstream signaling cascades, modulating gene expression involved in **cell proliferation, angiogenesis, and inflammation control**.

Interaction of PDRNs with A2 Receptors: PDRNs are short DNA fragments that, upon administration, are enzymatically degraded into nucleotides and nucleosides, including **adenosine and adenosine-like metabolites**. Adenosine is a natural ligand for adenosine receptors, and these metabolites can **activate A2 receptors**, particularly A2A, on target cells such as fibroblasts and endothelial cells. Some studies suggest that PDRN-derived fragments can **directly mimic adenosine**, binding to the A2A receptor and triggering its signaling pathways. Additionally, PDRNs may **increase local adenosine availability** by promoting nucleotide salvage pathways and reducing adenosine breakdown, thereby sustaining receptor activation and enhancing regenerative effects.

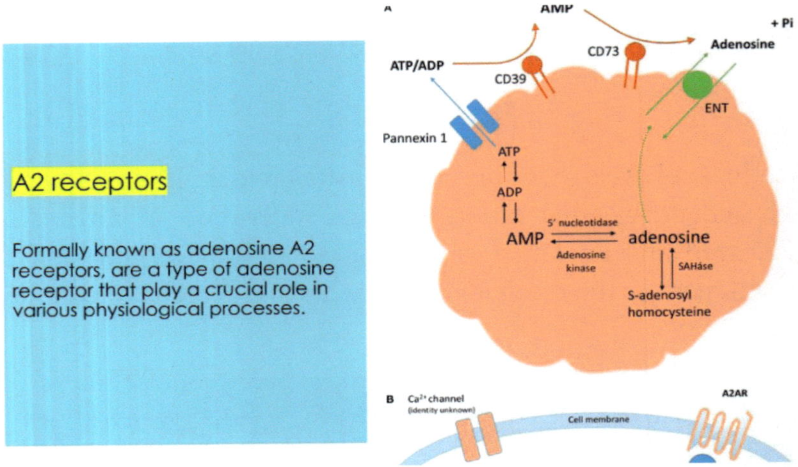

Upon **A2A receptor stimulation**, intracellular **cAMP levels rise in fibroblasts**, triggering enhanced **cell proliferation, collagen synthesis, and extracellular matrix (ECM) remodeling**. This mechanism is central to how **PDRNs accelerate wound healing and skin rejuvenation**. Activation of A2A receptors also upregulates key growth factors, such as **VEGF (Vascular Endothelial Growth Factor)**, promoting **angiogenesis** and improving microcirculation. Enhanced blood flow ensures better **oxygen and nutrient delivery**, further supporting tissue repair and regeneration.

Immunomodulatory Effects: Adenosine receptor activation can **downregulate pro-inflammatory cytokines** (e.g., TNF-α, IL-1β) while **upregulating anti-inflammatory mediators**, creating a balanced immune environment. This reduces tissue damage, limits excessive inflammation, and fosters optimal conditions for regeneration.

Nucleotide Salvage Synergy: PDRNs provide **nucleotide precursors** for DNA replication and repair in rapidly dividing cells. Coupled with **A2A-induced signaling**, this synergy accelerates **granulation tissue formation, re-epithelialization, and overall wound closure**.

Applications in Regenerative and Aesthetic Medicine: PDRN treatments—commonly **injected or applied topically to wound or treatment sites**—leverage A2 receptor signaling to **shorten healing timelines, reduce scarring, and enhance tissue quality**. In aesthetic applications, targeting fibroblasts via **A2A receptors** boosts collagen production, promotes skin regeneration, improves firmness, and diminishes wrinkles. By **modulating inflammation and enhancing vascularization**, PDRNs support faster recovery from procedures like **microneedling, laser therapy, or chemical peels**.

Chronic Wound Healing: The **angiogenic and anti-inflammatory properties** of A2 receptor activation are particularly valuable for conditions such as **chronic ulcers or diabetic wounds**, where impaired circulation and persistent inflammation impede healing.

In summary, **PDRNs (Polydeoxyribonucleotides)** exert regenerative effects by interacting with **A2A adenosine receptors** on fibroblasts, endothelial cells, and other target cells. Enzymatic degradation of PDRNs generates **adenosine-like metabolites** that elevate cAMP via A2 receptor signaling. This cascade stimulates **cell proliferation, angiogenesis, ECM remodeling, and anti-inflammatory responses**, bridging **nucleotide salvage with adenosine-mediated cellular communication** and delivering broad **tissue repair and aesthetic benefits**.

3. Anti-inflammatory Properties: Polynucleotides exhibit anti-inflammatory effects, which can help reduce swelling and redness, particularly after cosmetic procedures. This property may contribute to a more rapid recovery and improved outcomes in skin rejuvenation treatments.

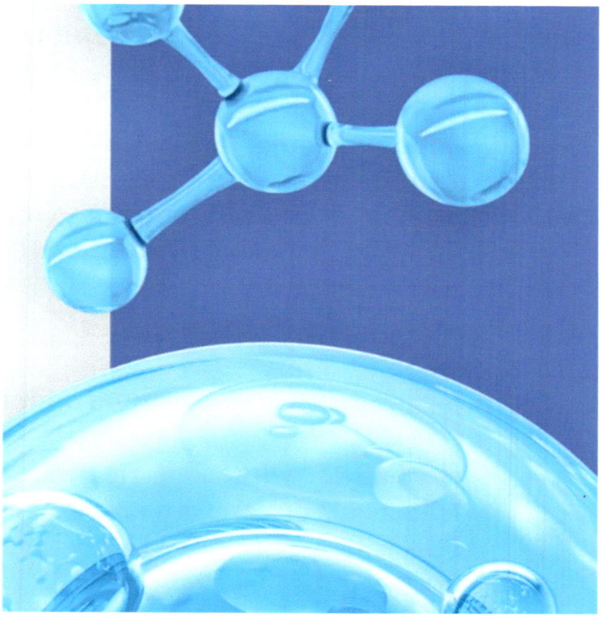

Q 39 – Tell me about inflammaging?

Inflammaging refers to a chronic, low-grade, systemic inflammatory state that develops with aging, contributing to age-related diseases and reduced cellular longevity. It is characterized by persistently elevated levels of **pro-inflammatory markers**—including cytokines such as **IL-6, TNF-α, and C-reactive protein (CRP)**—in the absence of overt infection. This state arises from cumulative stressors that disrupt **immune homeostasis**, including mitochondrial dysfunction, senescent cell accumulation, and dysregulated cellular signaling.

The term "**inflammaging**," a blend of *inflammation* and *aging*, captures this persistent, subclinical inflammatory condition that occurs naturally with age. It reflects an **imbalance between pro-inflammatory and anti-inflammatory processes**, leading to chronic tissue damage, impaired repair mechanisms, and heightened susceptibility to disease.

Key Features of Inflammaging:

- **Low-grade, chronic elevation** of inflammatory mediators such as **IL-1β, IL-6, and TNF-α**.
- **Association with age-related conditions**, including **cardiovascular disease, Alzheimer's disease, type 2 diabetes, and sarcopenia**.
- **Acceleration of cellular senescence**, impairing tissue repair, regenerative capacity, and overall cellular longevity.

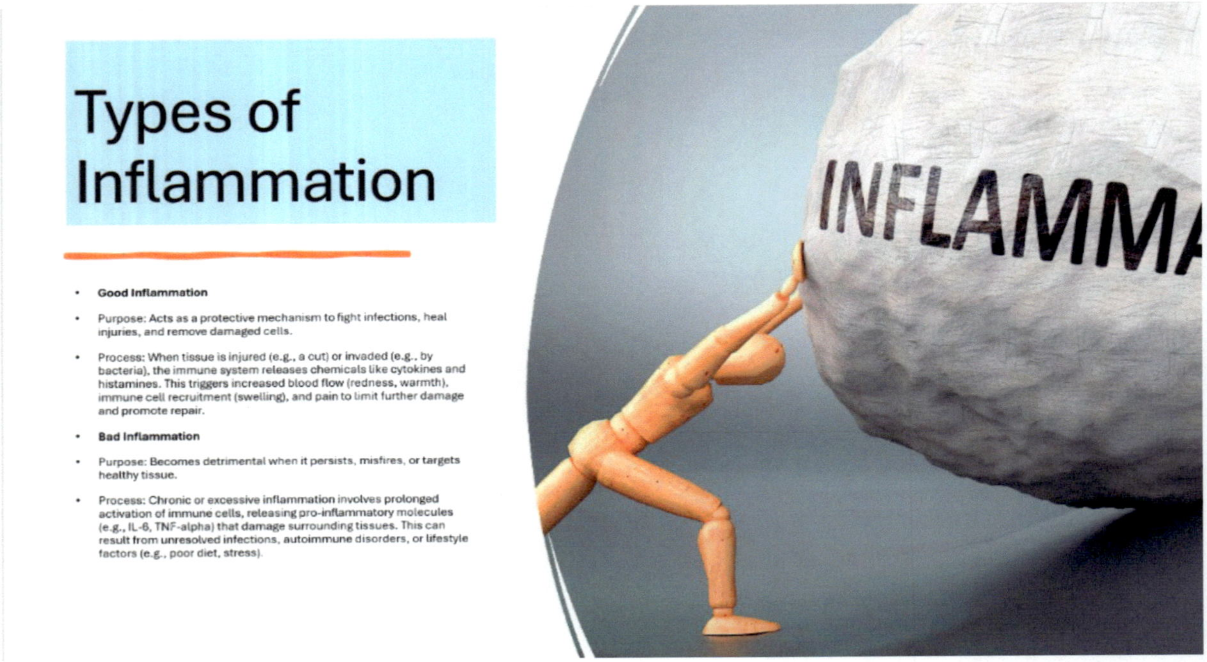

The Central Role of Inflammation

Let's start with a critical concept: inflammaging, the chronic, low-grade inflammation that drives ageing and disease. If we look at the top 15 causes of death in Europe—cardiovascular disease, cancer, stroke, diabetes, respiratory diseases, and more—14 of them are underpinned by inflammation. Acute inflammation is our body's hero, rushing in to fight infections or repair injuries. But chronic inflammation? It's a smoldering fire, silently damaging tissues, organs, and, most critically, the brain.

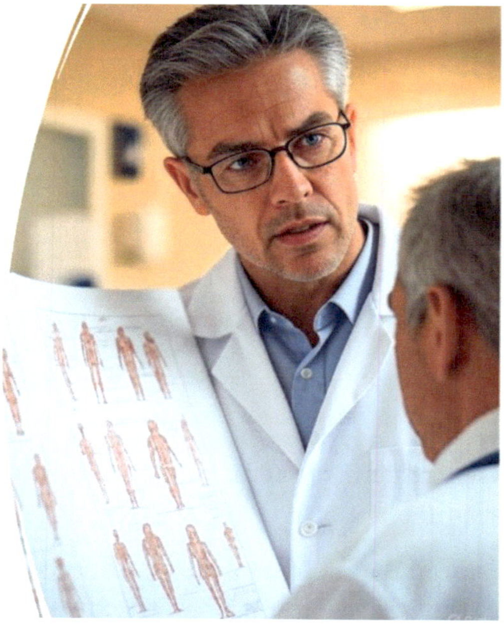

Mechanisms of Inflammaging

1. **Cellular Senescence:** Aging cells enter a senescent state and adopt a **senescence-associated secretory phenotype (SASP)**, releasing pro-inflammatory molecules such as **IL-6, IL-1β, and chemokines**. These secretions amplify both **local and systemic inflammation**, contributing to tissue dysfunction and the progression of age-related diseases.
2. **Mitochondrial Dysfunction:** Age-related mitochondrial damage leads to increased production of **reactive oxygen species (ROS)**, which activate inflammatory pathways—most notably **NF-κB signaling**—and stimulate the release of additional pro-inflammatory cytokines.
3. **Immune Dysregulation: Immunosenescence**, the gradual decline in immune competence, impairs the clearance of pathogens and senescent or damaged cells. Simultaneously, inflammaging drives **hyperactive innate immune responses**, such as chronic macrophage activation, further sustaining systemic inflammation.
4. **Accumulation of Damaged Biomolecules:** Proteins, DNA, and lipids damaged by oxidative stress or other insults accumulate with age, activating **inflammasomes** (e.g., **NLRP3**). This triggers the production of potent inflammatory cytokines such as **IL-1β and IL-18**, perpetuating tissue inflammation.
5. **Gut Dysbiosis:** Age-related alterations in the **gut microbiota** increase intestinal permeability ("leaky gut"), allowing bacterial components such as **lipopolysaccharides (LPS)** to enter circulation and exacerbate systemic inflammatory responses.
6. **Dysregulated Chemical Signaling:** Inflammaging involves **imbalances in cytokine, chemokine, and growth factor signaling**, disrupting normal cellular communication. For example, excessive **IL-6 signaling** can impair tissue repair and regeneration, in contrast to regenerative signals provided by **exosomes, secretomes, or neuroplasticity-enhancing interventions**.

Implications for Aging and Disease

Chronic, low-grade inflammation progressively degrades the **extracellular matrix (ECM)**, impairs **stem cell function**, and promotes **fibrosis**, collectively reducing tissue and organ functionality. Inflammaging is a major risk factor for numerous age-related diseases, including:

- **Neurodegenerative disorders** such as Alzheimer's disease, where chronic neuroinflammation contributes to neuronal loss.
- **Cardiovascular diseases**, including atherosclerosis, driven by persistent endothelial inflammation.
- **Metabolic disorders**, such as type 2 diabetes, where systemic inflammation exacerbates insulin resistance.

Additionally, inflammaging accelerates **telomere shortening** and cellular senescence, shortening cell lifespan and diminishing regenerative potential. Targeting inflammatory processes, particularly **senescence-associated secretory phenotype (SASP)** components, has been shown to extend **healthspan** and improve tissue resilience.

Therapeutic Strategies

Several interventions can mitigate inflammaging and its downstream effects:

- **Bioactive compounds:** Molecules like **resveratrol** (a sirtuin activator) and **cannabidiol (CBD)** suppress pro-inflammatory cytokine production and reduce oxidative stress.
- **Exosome-based therapies:** Exosomes can deliver **anti-inflammatory microRNAs or therapeutic agents** to senescent cells, modulating SASP and promoting tissue repair.
- **Lifestyle interventions:** Regular **exercise**, **caloric restriction**, and adherence to anti-inflammatory diets, such as the **Mediterranean diet**, effectively lower circulating levels of **IL-6, TNF-α, and CRP**, mitigating the effects of chronic inflammation.

Collectively, these strategies aim to **restore immune balance, reduce chronic inflammation, and preserve tissue function**, addressing the core mechanisms of inflammaging.

Prof. Dr. Patrick Treacy honoured with Lifetime Achievement Awards at the ZYLAN Congress

August 2024 – The ZYLAN Congress honored Prof. Dr. Patrick Treacy and Prof. Yang Rong Ya with Lifetime Achievement Awards, celebrating their outstanding contributions and pioneering impact in the fields of aesthetic medicine and dermatology.

Prof. Yang Rong Ya

Chief Physician and Director of Dermatology at the PLA General Hospital in Beijing, Prof. Yang serves as Vice President of the China Plastic and Aesthetic Association and Chair of the Dermatology and Venereal Disease Prevention and Control Branch of the Chinese Preventive Medicine Association. She also leads the PLA Dermatology Committee, acts as Executive Deputy Director of the Chinese Medical Beauty Training Project, and serves as Executive Director of the Beijing Medical Association. Her leadership spans clinical, academic, and professional spheres, cementing her influence in dermatology and aesthetic medicine across China.

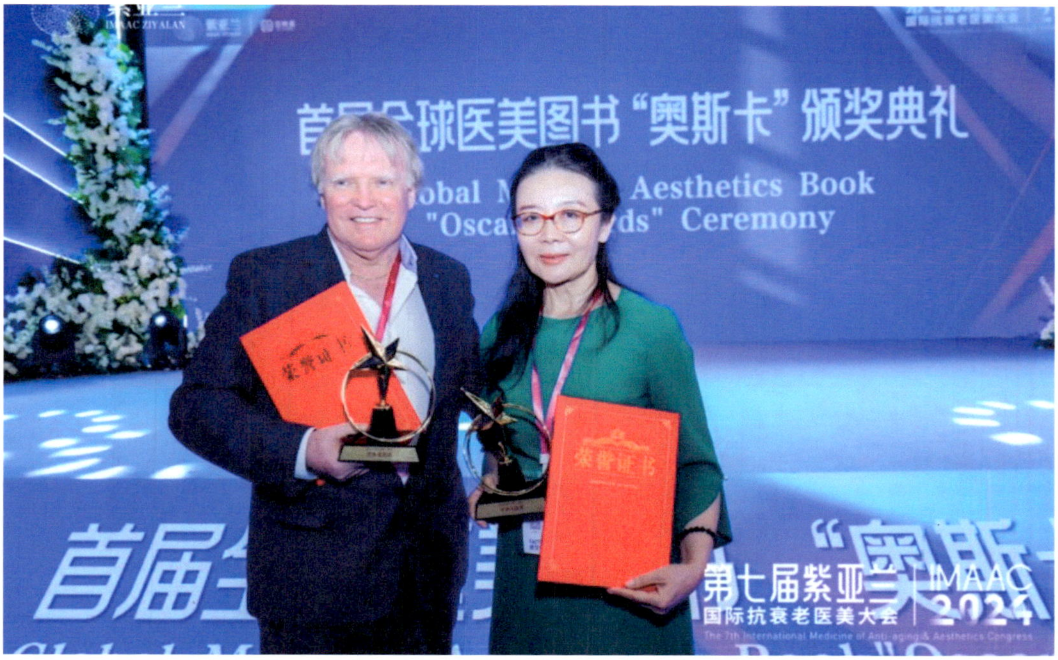

Prof. Dr. Patrick Treacy

A best-selling author and internationally acclaimed leader in aesthetic medicine, Prof. Dr. Treacy has received numerous awards recognizing his pioneering contributions to the field. He serves as Visiting Professor of Dermatology at Isra University in Pakistan and holds a Fellowship in

Cosmetic Surgery and Medicine from the Australian College, a Laureate in Aesthetic Medicine from the Azerbaijan College, and the CMME medal from the Mexican College.

In 2024, Prof. Dr. Treacy was honored with the “Man of the Year Award” in Ireland. Previously, he was named the “Top Aesthetic Practitioner in the World” at the MyFaceMyBody Global Awards in Las Vegas (2019). He has also been recognized multiple times as “Doctor of the Year” in the UK and Ireland. His Ailesbury Clinic has earned the distinction of “Top Clinic in Ireland” five times over the past seven years, reflecting his sustained excellence in clinical practice and patient care.

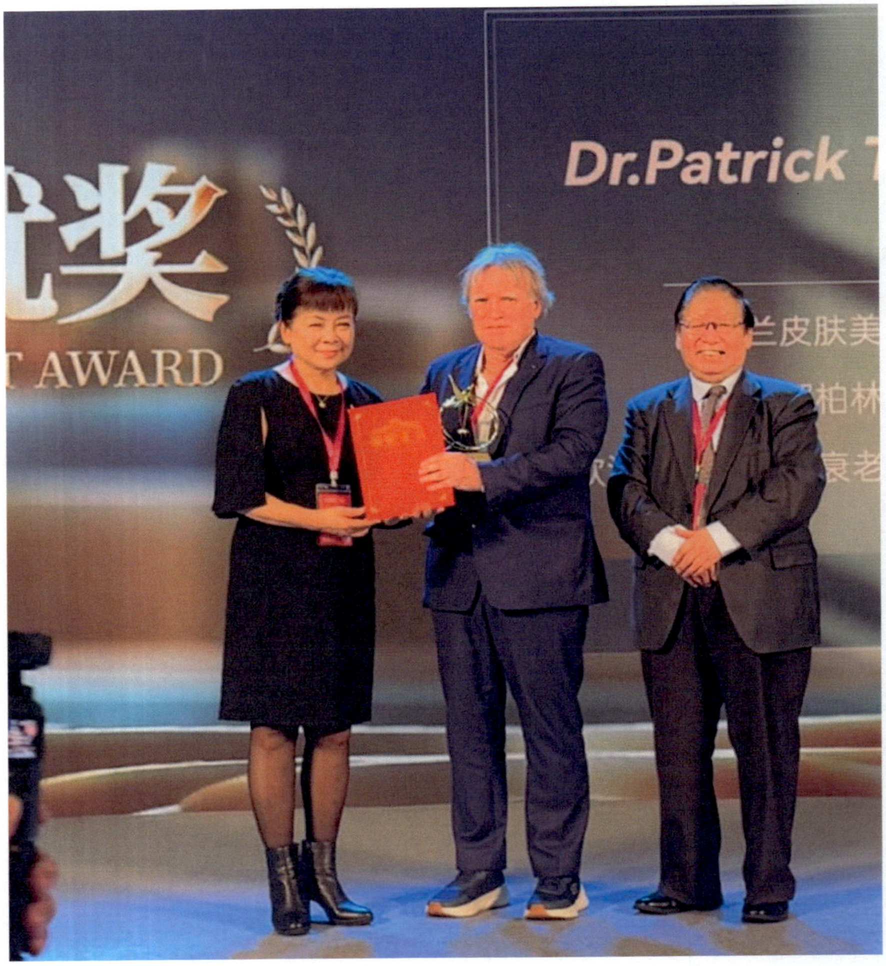

These Lifetime Achievement Awards from the ZYLAN Congress highlight the enduring contributions of both Prof. Dr. Patrick Treacy and Prof. Yang Rong Ya in advancing modern aesthetic medicine and dermatology, setting new benchmarks for clinical excellence, innovation, and patient care.

His innovative research has significantly advanced patient safety, particularly through the development of hyaluronidase protocols in aesthetic medicine. Internationally celebrated for his work with stem cells, platelet-rich plasma, and growth signaling factors, Prof. Dr. Treacy has successfully treated necrosis following vascular occlusion. He has been awarded the AMEC Trophy on three occasions (in Paris and Monaco) and has received multiple MyFaceMyBody awards. In addition, he has chaired the Organising Committee for the Royal Society of Medicine Aesthetic Congress and led the Irish Association of Cosmetic Doctors, serves on the editorial boards of several international journals, and has trained over 10,000 healthcare professionals worldwide earning the title of "Top International Aesthetic Trainer 2023" in Karachi, Pakistan.

His innovative research has significantly advanced patient safety, particularly through the development of hyaluronidase protocols in aesthetic medicine. Internationally recognized for his expertise with stem cells, platelet-rich plasma, and growth signaling factors, Prof. Dr. Treacy has successfully managed complications such as necrosis following vascular occlusion. He has been awarded the AMEC Trophy on three occasions in Paris and Monaco and has received multiple MyFaceMyBody awards.

In addition to his clinical achievements, he has chaired the Organising Committee for the Royal Society of Medicine Aesthetic Congress, led the Irish Association of Cosmetic Doctors, served on the editorial boards of several international journals, and trained over 10,000 healthcare professionals worldwide, earning the title of "Top International Aesthetic Trainer 2023" in Karachi, Pakistan.

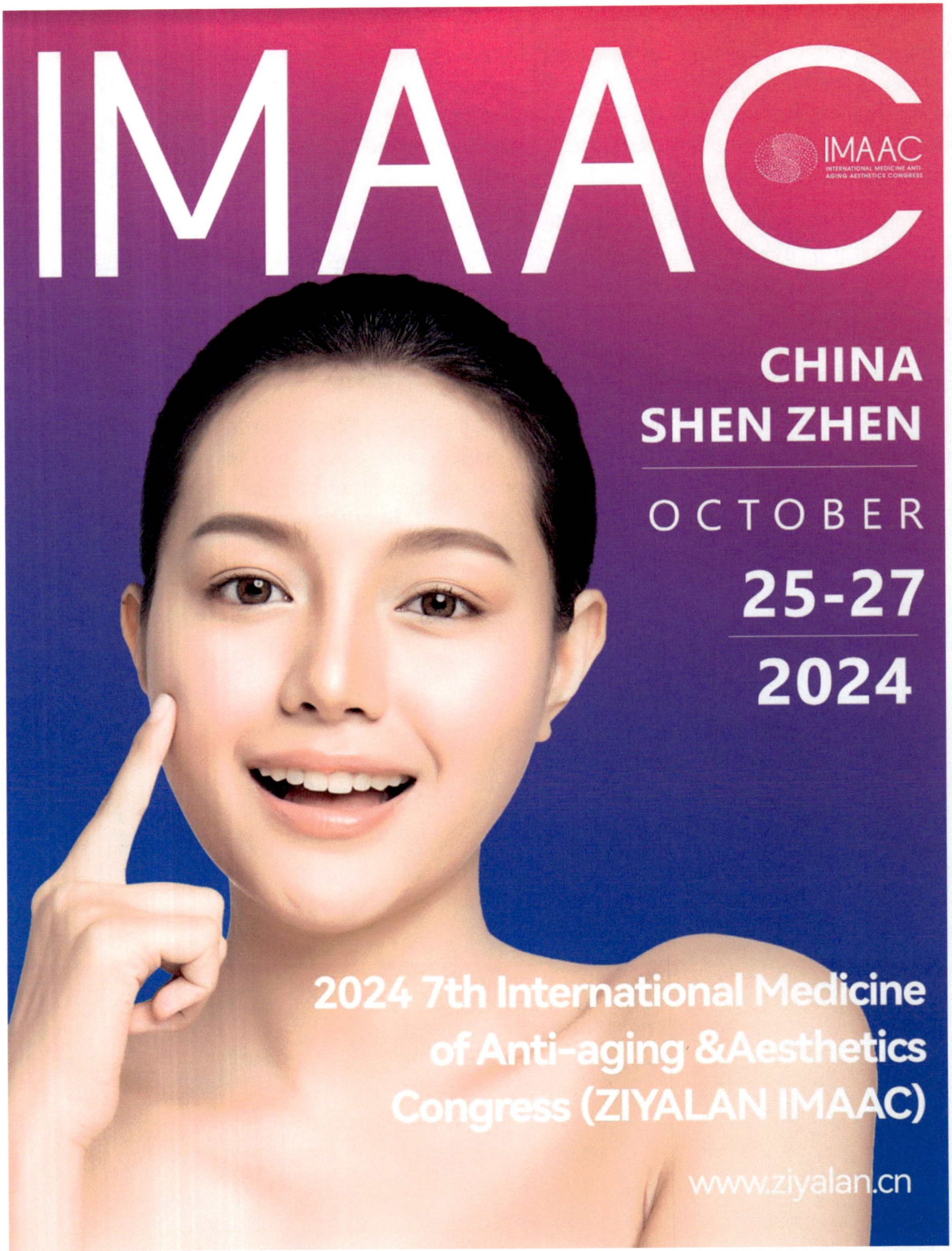
IMAAC
IMAAC
INTERNATIONAL MEDICINE ANTI-AGING AESTHETICS CONGRESS
CHINA
SHEN ZHEN
OCTOBER
25-27
2024
2024 7th International Medicine of Anti-aging &Aesthetics Congress (ZIYALAN IMAAC)
www.ziyalan.cn

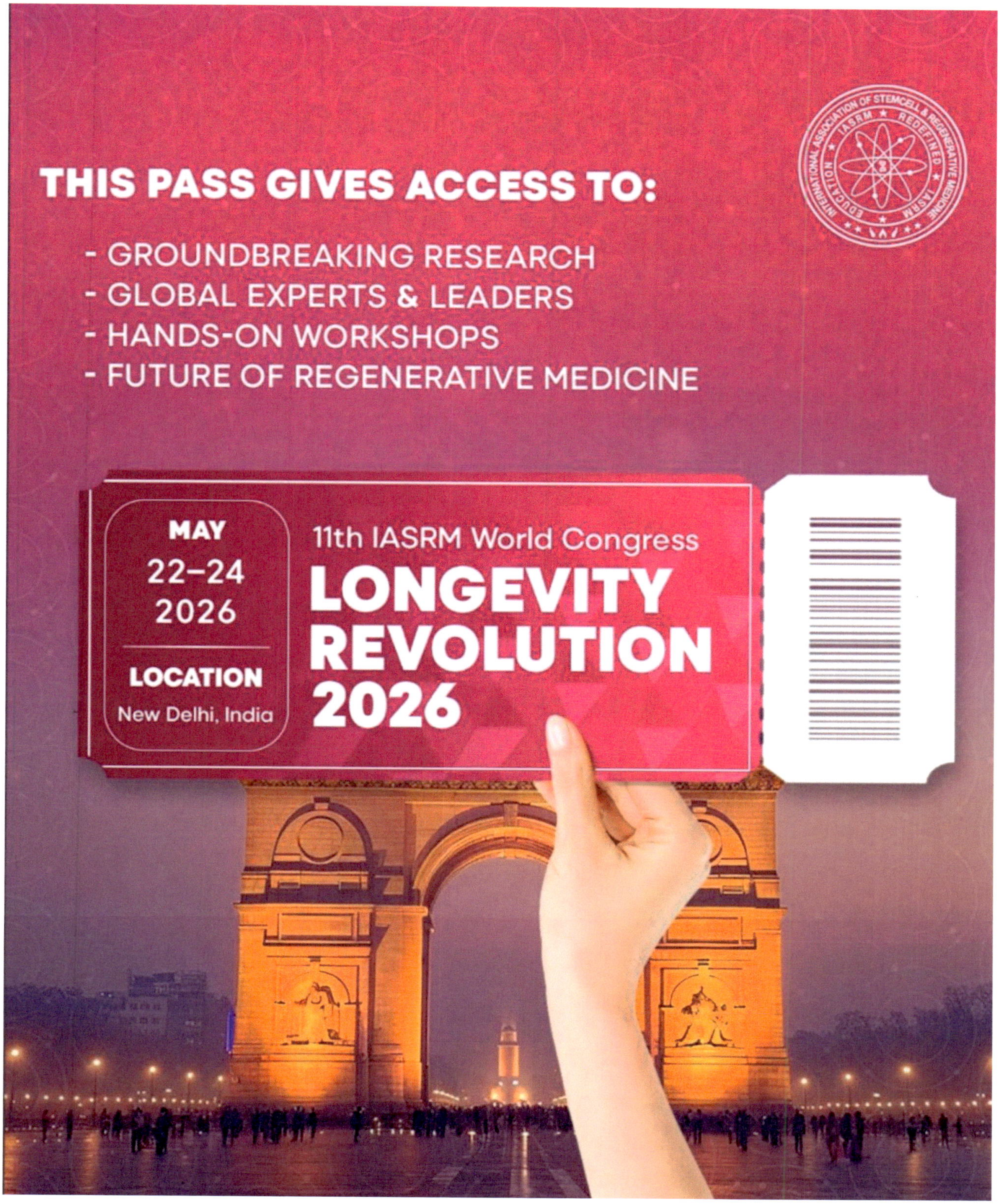

THIS PASS GIVES ACCESS TO:
- GROUNDBREAKING RESEARCH
- GLOBAL EXPERTS & LEADERS
- HANDS-ON WORKSHOPS
- FUTURE OF REGENERATIVE MEDICINE
INTERNATIONAL ASSOCIATION OF STEMCELL & REGENERATIVE MEDICINE
IASRM
REDEFINED
EDUCATION
MAY
22–24
2026
LOCATION
New Delhi, India
11th IASRM World Congress
LONGEVITY
REVOLUTION
2026

Prof Patrick Treacy Awards (2023-2025)

- **Winner – World Regenerative Medicine Innovation Award for NS Hair Growth (London) 2025**
- **Winner – Top Aesthetic Clinic in Ireland. (Dublin, Ireland) 2025**
- **Winner – Lifetime Achievement Award for advances in Aesthetic Medicine (Milan, Italy) 2025**
- **Winner – Lifetime Achievement Award for advances in Aesthetic Medicine (Shenzhen, China) 2024**
- **Winner – Lifetime Achievement Award for advances in Aesthetic Medicine (Cork, Ireland) 2024**
- **Winner – IMCAS China Award for Dedication to Science, Medicine and Patients (Shanghai) 2025**
- **Winner – Private Healthcare Excellence Award 'Best Aesthetic Clinic in Ireland' (Belfast) 2025**
- **Winner – Top Aesthetic Clinic in Ireland. (Cork, Ireland) 2024**
- **Winner – 'Man of the Year' (Ireland) for Humanitarianism in Africa (Cork) 2024**
- **Winner – Recognition of Excellence and Outstanding Contribution to Medicine (Dubai, UAE) 2024**
- **Winner – Top Aesthetic Clinic in Ireland. (Cork, Ireland) 2024**
- **Winner – Top Global Pioneer in Aesthetic Medicine (Dublin, Ireland) 2024**
- **Winner – Top UK & Ireland Aesthetic Clinic (London, UK) 2024**
- **Winner – Top UK & Ireland Aesthetic Doctor (London, UK) 2024**
- **Winner – Top Aesthetic Clinic in Ireland (Dublin, Ireland) 2023**
- **Winner – Top Irish Aesthetic Doctor (Dublin, Ireland) 2023**
- **Winner – Top Global Master Trainer in Aesthetic Medicine (Karachi, Pakistan) 2023**
- **Winner – PAADS Award 'Outstanding Contributions to Aesthetic Medicine (Karachi, Pakistan) 2023**
- **Winner – Irish Healthcare Centre Award 'Best Aesthetic Clinic in Ireland' (Dublin) 2023**

- **Winner – GHP Global Excellence Award 'Best Aesthetic Clinic in Ireland' (London) 2023**
- **Winner – Tia Maria 'Lifetime Achievement Award' (Cork, Ireland) 2023**
- **Winner – Tia Maria 'Top Aesthetic Doctor in Ireland' (Cork, Ireland) 2023**

Prof Patrick Treacy Awards (2017-2023)

- **Winner – AIDA Trophy 'Outstanding Contributions to Aesthetic Medicine (Abu Dhabi, UAE) May 2022**
- **Winner – MyFaceMyBody 'Top Global Medical Practitioner' 2019 (Las Vegas, USA) November 2019**
- **Winner – MyFaceMyBody 'Top UK & Ire Medical Practitioner' 2019 (Las Vegas, USA) November 2019**
- **Winner – AMEC Anti-aging & Beauty Trophy 'Best Global Clinical Case' (Monaco), October 2019**
- **Winner – Irish Healthcare Award 'Best Medical Aesthetic Clinic (Dublin, Ireland), Sept 2019**
- **Winner – MyFaceMyBody 'Scientific Contributions to the Aesthetic Industry' (London), March 2018**
- **Winner – Irish Healthcare Award 'Best Medical Research Award' (Dublin, Ireland), March 2017**
- **Winner – MyFaceMyBody Award 'Ultimate 100 Global Aesthetic Leaders' (Los Angeles), August 2017**
- **Winner – British College of Aesthetic Medicine 'Research Award' (London, UK) September 2017**

Made in the USA
Monee, IL
26 June 2026

55822805R00093